GETTING BACK TO GOOD

10 Steps to Be the Change You Wish to See

Ken Ferrara

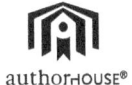

authorHOUSE®

AuthorHouse™
1663 Liberty Drive, Suite 200
Bloomington, IN 47403
www.authorhouse.com
Phone: 1-800-839-8640

First published by AuthorHouse   7/2/2008

ISBN: 978-1-4343-9829-1 (sc)

Printed in the United States of America
Bloomington, Indiana

This book is printed on acid-free paper.

~ A Tale of Two Wolves ~

One evening an old Cherokee told his grandson about a battle that goes on inside people. He said, "My son, the battle is between two wolves inside us all. The first wolf is evil. It is anger, envy, jealousy, sorrow, regret, greed, arrogance, self-pity, guilt, resentment, inferiority, lies, false pride, superiority, and ego.

The second wolf is good. It is joy, peace, love, hope, serenity, humility, kindness, benevolence, empathy, generosity, truth, compassion, and faith." The grandson thought about it for a moment and then asked his grandfather, "Which wolf wins?" The old Cherokee simply replied, "The one you feed."

—Author unknown.

CONTENTS

PREFACE

"You must be the change you wish to see in the world."

-Mahatma Gandhi

This profound quote holds answers to the riddles of world peace, environmental issues, eliminating world hunger and suffering, and creating more care and compassion in our world. While that is a lot to ask from a group of twelve words, those same words have even more influence — unlocking gates of fulfillment and happiness in your life. They open doors to better health, improved relationships, attitudes of gratitude, becoming more patient and selfless, as well as finding purpose.

On the surface, Gandhi's insights may seem warm, fuzzy, and well intentioned, but once we get down to brass tacks, do they lack real-world practicality? After all, what can one person do to bring about change? Well, the answer may surprise you. Consider a variation of Gandhi's quote; "You must be the change you need in your life in order to be the change you wish to see in our world." Good, positive, beneficial changes you make — becoming healthier, treating others better, and improving your outlook, will enhance your life in many ways and encourage you to share goodness.

I would venture to say that many, if not most people believe our world is not as good as it could be. If this is how you feel, as I do, it's important to recognize that you and I have the power to change that fact. Start by taking a step back from all aspects of your daily routine to see what and where you can improve, and start thinking about how you can make your difference — in your life and just as importantly, in the lives of others.

We all have our good moments, and dare I say, less than stellar times, but I think it's safe to say most of us could find ways to live a better life. Do I have things I need to work on? Sure! (Ask my wife or kids, and I'm sure they could draw up a nice long list.) However, when I observe myself, I wear the proverbial 'rose-colored glasses' and think I'm a little better than I actually am. I don't necessarily see areas where I can improve or how I am selfish, unhealthy, indifferent, or even hurtful to others. That's why it's important to delve deep into daily habits, routines, and thoughts to see what needs work. Also, asking others who know you well can really open your eyes to what needs changing, but we'll get to that later.

Plenty of opportunities to think and act with more goodness in every aspect of life present themselves everyday. From talking to a family member or friend you have not spoken with for years to simply letting that car pull out in front of you; from living a healthy lifestyle to maintaining a positive perspective, you can make good choices that will bring immense benefits to you and yours.

Speaking of being positive, imagine for a moment that a kitchen table is in front of you, and on that table is a glass filled exactly halfway to the top with water. If you ask different people to describe what they see, you will get three profoundly different answers. The first description, which is optimistic, positive, and cheerful, is that the glass is half-full (maybe even overflowing!). With this perspective, the glass has plenty of water; you can enjoy it, share it with others, and feel good about it. The second description is a little on the pessimistic side — stating that the glass is half-empty. This makes you worry if there will be enough water, so you don't share as much as you should and constantly think about having enough. The third description, the most negative of the bunch is, "What glass are you talking about? I don't see a glass."

What does that glass of water look like to you? On the full side? On the empty side? Or, "What glass?" As life brings blessings and trials, I'm sure each of us describes our own "glass of water" in each of those ways, I know I certainly have.

Is it possible for someone to be positive all the time? Of course not, we are human, and we all have moments we may be less than proud of; and let's face it, we'll probably have more. However, having said that, I want to firmly impress upon you that we — you and I, and everyone we know — have the power to make a positive difference in our own lives as well as in our greater world.

Questioning if you can become a better person in today's hectic, sometimes-unforgiving world is natural. Have you ever thought, "I am so busy caring for my responsibilities that I just don't have time right now, I will get to it when I am better off." Or what about, "Things are so messed up, busy, and difficult nowadays, can I really bring about change and make a difference?" *Absolutely*! And there are powerful reasons to do just that.

Despite the cliché, living with goodness becomes its own, fantastic reward, on a personal level as well as on a grand scale. Actively seeking to become a better person for yourself and others around you will move you toward a more positive and enriching life.

Are you ready to:

➢ Find more happiness and a peaceful sense of fulfillment;

➢ Deal with situations and your relationships more positively, with abundant patience;

➢ Constantly remember what you should be thankful for, from your health to your family and friends to nature, even the day itself;

➢ Show tolerance of the dynamic diversity in our world, from the multitude of differing spiritual beliefs to widely varying personal views and appearances;

➢ Care for yourself physically, emotionally, and spiritually;

➢ Mend broken or faltering relationships;

➢ Show more kindness and gratitude, even through the challenging circumstances life inevitably brings;

➢ Offer apologies and forgiveness to those you have hurt, as well as to those who've hurt you;

➢ Find meaning and purpose for life by learning to live for more than yourself;

➢ Realize peace of mind.

These points will become reality for you when you choose to think positively and take ACTion.

By the fact that you are reading this now, I know you believe in your ability to make a difference. While you may not have had total success in the past with relationships, your health, a career, or in being a selfless person, today you can *begin anew*. You have taken that first, symbolic step, now it's time to start walking.

I optimistically believe in the positive potential of the human spirit. As you read on, I hope you become inspired to wholeheartedly care for others and view life with a glass half-full (hopefully overflowing) perspective, and consider these thought provoking questions. Who am I? Who do I want to be? How can I make my difference? What am I meant to do with my life?

Another big question is, "Am I truly happy and fulfilled?" Not in the sense that you have visited those places you've dreamt about, climbed the corporate ladder, or achieved your goals. No, what I'm talking about is the fulfillment that comes from knowing you have done your best to be the change you want to see in your life and in our world. To know you have fulfilled your purpose here so completely with respect to caring for yourself, others, and embracing goodness, that if you lay your head down for the last time tonight, you could truly rest, find peace, and know your life matters.

Apply the simple, yet powerful lessons and concepts you'll find here to all aspects of life; whether that's as a parent, a caring person, a student, a family member, or a friend; as a teacher, a religious/spiritual leader and follower, an employee, the head of a company, or the head of a nation. Use this book as a tool to improve personal relationships, attitudes, and perspectives, and on a grand scale toward helping achieve more harmony in our world. The sky's the limit when you decide to be the change and feed your good wolf.

CHAPTER 1

GETTING BACK TO GOOD

"All people have a basic decency and goodness. If they listen to it and act on it, they are giving a great deal of what it is the world needs most. It is not complicated, but it takes courage. It takes courage for people to listen to their own good."

—Pablo Casals

At times, this world seems to be declining at an ever-increasing rate. 'Going down the tubes' is what my grandma used to say. From vast amounts of negativity, selfishness, and violence that are so readily observable by turning on the news or picking up a paper, to failing relationships, health problems, human suffering, financial troubles, and frightening personal and global issues; one could say my grandma was on the right track.

Problems facing us today seem so daunting and unapproachable, that feeling helpless and hopeless to affect any sort of real, positive change can be a natural reaction. Sometimes day-to-day life seems so hard, demanding, and unfair, that you may have little time, ambition, or energy for being a selfless and giving person. Taking care of your needs exclusively may even feel like a requirement for survival, so why should you strive to live with more goodness?

While no laws of humanity dictate that you must be patient, generous, accepting, or kind, you have the choice to a live a life full of selfishness and negativity, or one that can be bursting with optimism, health, purpose, and clarity. What will be your choice?

⁓ **What is getting back to good?** ⁓

Here's the short answer: Getting back to good is a process that can transform your attitudes, health, and perspective by helping you focus positively in thought and action. For instance, are you as healthy you could be? If not, you can become inspired to make choices to correct that. Are there some relationships that could be better in your life? If so, discover what part you play keeping those relationships from being as good as they could be (and trust me, we all play a part). Do your goals seem unattainable? They're not; you must simply learn to incorporate goodness into those goals and they can be realized in due time. Do you have faith? In yourself…in humanity…in goodness? Like that snippet of wisdom from the old Cherokee, "Which wolf wins? The one you feed." By feeding your 'good wolf,' you can effectively bring about immensely powerful, beneficial, and positive changes to your life.

This process shows you why striving toward individual goodness for yourself, as well as for others around you is essential, and provides guided, practical steps to achieve these goals. "To-Do" checklists create inspiring visual aids and provide tangible direction on how to effectively apply these concepts in everyday life. There are also note pages and a journal to help chart your progress and plan.

Fortunately, this process is customizable to fit your life by the person who knows that life best — you! Identifying and applying positive attitudes and actions through your particular beliefs and values will effectively help you address and attack negativity. By choosing to live with more selflessness and patience, make healthy choices, and encourage happiness, you will naturally become a more tolerant, giving, and fulfilled person.

I realize that changing for the better can seem overwhelming and challenging, but simple, powerful steps can help you enhance and improve aspects of your life — one step at a time, one day at a time. Some concepts here are designed to simply be a starting point of awareness for you to find more health, happiness, and gratitude, while other tips and techniques can be put into action today with immediate, positive results. You can also follow up with resources on the web and recommended reading to help you apply individual concepts in a more detailed and personalized manner.

Will you be able to fix problems in your life by getting back to good? Yes, many troubles, problems, and day-to-day inconveniences can be thoroughly resolved if you make an honest effort to apply the principles and procedures on these pages. You may find that many challenges facing you are actually caused by, ready for this — you. Yes, by your thoughts and actions. For example, do you treat people as you want to be treated? How do you deal with adversity? Do you take care of yourself as you should? Are you a persistent optimist, or constant pessimist? Are you a person who wallows in self-pity when life doesn't go your way, or do you accentuate the positives?

When life gets tough, as it certainly can, tend to your challenges by doing what is necessary to fix them, but do so with the care, compassion, and positive attitudes emphasized here. Your perspective can change from one of "What about me?" or "My way is the only way," to one of overwhelming care and concern for others. Remember, this process is not an immediate solution for the troubles and problems of an individual life or for the problems of our world, but simply because it may not be immediate, does not mean it isn't worthwhile. Becoming the change you need in your life in order to live with more goodness is one of the best things you can do with your precious time here.

Getting back to good is not reserved for those who have committed crimes, lived extremely selfishly, or committed illegal or immoral actions. And while it may be easy to go through a list of people in your mind who you think need this book more than you, please try your best to keep the focus on yourself. Spiritual, good-natured, and caring people can treat others (as well as themselves) with less kindness, generosity, respect, and tolerance than possible. Fortunately, most people exhibit negative or "bad" thoughts and actions that are relatively minor in scope, and require subtle changes in attitude and action to get back to good

All of this sounds good in theory, I know, but in order for it to make a difference in your life, there is going to have to be some honest effort, reflection, planning, and of course action, on your part. Your attitude, and what you do on a daily basis with that attitude will be the driver and catalyst for changes you will see. How successful can you be? Consider this:

Who am I?

"I am your constant companion. I will push you forward to success or I will drag you down to failure. I am completely at your command. 80% of what you do, you might as well hand over to me, I will do it promptly, and I will do it correctly.

I am easily managed; you must merely be firm with me. Show me what you'd like to have done, and after a couple of lessons, I will do it automatically. I am the servant of all great people. Alas, I am the servant of all failures as well. All who are great, I have made great. All who are failures, I have made failures.

I am not a machine; but I do work with the precision of a machine and the intellect of a human. Take me, train me, be firm with me, and I'll lay the world at your feet. Be easy with me, and I will destroy you!" Who am I? I am your habits!

-Author Unknown

No matter what is written in this book (or any book for that matter), how well it makes sense, or how good it sounds, you are ultimately in control of how effective it will be. Now take a moment, smile, and enjoy your ride…!

~The Big Picture~

Before beginning your personal journey, let's take a moment and look at the big picture to see how each of us connects to everyone and everything through our common responsibility to live with goodness. Then, we can move onto the process of getting back to good, and finally start implementing tips and techniques to be the change you want to see in your life, and start sharing that goodness with the world.

"Today, more than ever, we need to make a fundamental recognition of the basic oneness of humanity, the foundation of our perspective on the world and its challenges. From the dangerous rate of global warming to the widening gap between rich and poor, from the rise of global terrorism to regional conflicts, we need a fundamental shift in our attitudes and our consciousness — a wider, more holistic outlook."

-The Dalai Lama

As we gaze at the dawn of a new millennium, it's easy to see humanity has gained vast amounts of knowledge and advanced technology. Today, we have more collective power at our disposal than ever before, and ideally, the world should be a nicer place. From the standpoint of our abilities and achievements, the world should be an abundant, safe, and caring place to live because we have the technical means and abilities to care for one another as at no other time in the past.

We have the capability to eradicate disease, feed the hungry, and make poverty history. While technological advancements and changes are empowering, humankind, to put it mildly, still has troubles. On a personal level, you can have problems with relationships, your health, and your perspective, or you may be selfish and angry about situations you encounter daily. Perhaps you feel hopeless at times – like life lacks meaning and purpose. On a global scale, countries wage war, there is immense, crushing poverty and famine around the world, and people continue trying to justify differences, rather than focusing on and embracing our common ties.

Human beings epitomize the very definition of goodness by loving, caring, giving selflessly, and showing compassion and tolerance toward one another, but the unfortunate reality is that, in many ways, the opposite is also true, as we act with varying degrees of immorality, selfishness, intolerance, and negativity.

Why are people selfish? How can we be rude and indifferent to others, simply caring for our own? Why are wars fought? What prompts some people to live a life of excess while so many others scrounge for food, health, and shelter every day? Why does one person believe his or her children, possessions, beliefs, or rights are more important than yours? Or vice versa? One simple answer is human nature — that's just the way we are, right?

Are the darker aspects of humanity simply problems of human nature? Where do these undesirable, negative thoughts and behaviors come from? What can be done to lessen their growth and slow or even stop their impact? These questions are not easily answered, but one truth remains constant — you can find answers and put them into practice in your life because you have the *choice* to think positively or negatively, and act accordingly.

Start by accepting what Gandhi profoundly stated, "You must be the change you wish to see in the world." Do you treat others with less kindness, patience, and tolerance than you could? Do you treat your body well, eating a healthy diet, exercising, lowering the amount of stress in your life, and finding quality time for you and yours? Do you only care for yourself by exclusively dealing with your needs, desires, and beliefs, leaving others to fend for themselves? Are you as generous and giving as you should be? As you could be? These questions are just the start. Search deeply in your life regarding your health, your family, your environment, and for ways you can make your difference.

~ Goodness ~

By basic definition, goodness is beneficial. This definition is inclusive and all encompassing, open to many diverse interpretations — not something exclusively associated with a single spiritual, cultural, or personal view. It is not overbearing or narrowly focused, and allows people to readily offer kindness, nurture tolerance and health, and exhibit selflessness.

Various cultures and individuals have diverse ideas and beliefs, inevitably leading to differing perspectives. While these different outlooks and views have inspired the closeness, co-operation, compassion, and care of the human spirit, they have also spawned separation, prejudice, intolerance, and hatred (ironically, often committed in the name of goodness).

For centuries, philosophers, theologians, and scholars have debated issues surrounding the true nature of goodness, but it is not as complex as we make it out to seem. Flow charts or thick books are not required for people to understand it. Sure, there are times when the meaning of goodness can and should be debated and discussed or philosophized. However, in my opinion, that happens much too often, causing the spirit of goodness to get muffled, complicated, and ignored. That's why *Getting Back to Good* doesn't center on unanswerable questions, complex philosophies, or separation and exclusion. Rather, it focuses on using our connectedness and commonalities to help bring more goodness into the world.

> *"The welfare of each is bound up in the welfare of all."*
> **—Helen Keller**

We share immense commonality as human beings. Before any race, physical difference, or creed, and before any nationality or mindset, each and every one of us is human — fundamentally common and equal. Who we are, what groups we belong to, or what we do for a living makes no difference, as we all travel over the same ocean called life. Of course, each of us is on a different type of ship, sailing a different course, but we ultimately travel to the same destination.

For all intents and purposes, we desire the same things from life: to fulfill our needs, to have the ability to love and care for ourselves and our loved ones, to have health, and to believe and connect to that which is important to us. Our commonalities dictate that we share life together. As such, the responsibility for living with goodness applies to all people equally, from the poor to the rich; from heads of state to followers and leaders of differing spiritual beliefs; from business and community leaders to famous, "powerful," and everyday people. Creed, culture, country, and social class, as well as variations in ideology, upbringing, or personality make no difference — everyone is subject to universal laws of goodness.

In the biggest possible picture, there is no "us against them," or "you against me," as we are all in this together. Obviously, you must provide and care for yourself, protect what is yours, and feel connected to people, beliefs, and systems, but in the end, one of the most crucial battles you will fight is to think and act with goodness toward yourself and others, as you are accountable for that.

By focusing on processes, complicated rules, and over-analyzed interpretations, rather than focusing time, resources, and energies on living with goodness, we are choosing to move away from it. When this happens, the profound simplicity of goodness — to foster and nurture the encouraging, beneficial aspects of life is minimized and ignored. While changing small things in your every day actions will not instantly bring about world peace, end world hunger, resolve that argument with your sister, or help you lose fifty pounds overnight, living with goodness is as necessary to your life as air. *All* thoughts and behaviors that are good make a positive difference.

~ Find Your Way ~

As an individual with unique views and styles, you will find and develop the path back to good on your own terms, in conjunction with your personal beliefs and values. The specific interpretation and implementation is for you to decide upon and incorporate in your own way; however, be careful not to concentrate on your interpretations so intensely that you forget to implement them.

Take small, steady steps and changes will come. As your thoughts, perspectives, and actions become more positive and encouraging, you will notice the world around you change. By taking part in this effort, you are directly responsible for bringing more goodness into our world. Your life can be better, and this world *will* be better, when you become as good as you can be.

One small but vitally important reminder: Do not let encounters with death or tragedies become your wake-up call. Change your thoughts, actions, and life now — don't wait until it's too late. Make amends for any wrongs you have caused and treat others with goodness not because you are forced to, but because it's the right thing to do. Find your way back to good.

"How lovely to think that no one need wait a moment, we can start now, start slowly changing the world. How lovely that everyone, great and small, can make their contribution…how we can always, always give something, if only kindness."

—Anne Frank

CHAPTER 2

THE PROCESS

It is not what they profess, but what
they practice that makes them good.

—Greek Proverb

Getting back to good is not as simple as saying, "practice what you preach," or "just be good." As human beings, we are very complex and easily affected by different situations and circumstances that constantly shape and mold our choices and actions. Just as the Greek proverb states, we can profess all we want, but where the rubber meets the road is what really counts.

Our inherent knowledge of goodness, whether that means being kind and compassionate with others, feeling awe-struck when looking up at the stars or standing next to the ocean, or knowing what is good and healthy for us, can only be applied by choice and effort. Much like a muscle, this knowledge must be used often in order to keep it functional and strong. When a muscle is not used, it becomes weak, frail, susceptible to damage, and unable to function properly. Similarly, when we do not choose to apply our innate wisdom of what is good, that sense becomes weak and unable to function as designed, giving way to negativity, selfishness, and unhealthy attitudes and outlooks.

Living with goodness is something you must choose with every decision because opportunities to make the right choices face you every day. With regard to health, do you walk up the stairs, or do you take the elevator? Will you make a healthy lunch choice today, or will you opt for that greasy burger and fries? Do you commit to actively move and train your body several times per week? Are you leading by example with your children and loved ones, or simply saying, "do as I say, not as I do."

When it comes to living with more patience and kindness, do you remain calm with your kids? Do you make time for family and friends? Are you reflecting on what you are given everyday? Do you make your difference? Does being patient in traffic accurately describe you, or are you 'less than proud' of your behavior behind the wheel? Finally, will you do your best to keep a positive outlook and see the abundant goodness in your world with an attitude of gratitude?

To help guide choices of goodness, some people find direction through spiritual and religious beliefs, while others rely on different motivations. Try not to complicate goodness with unnecessary details, complex guidelines, or principles of segregation and superiority. Rather, encourage your inherent knowledge, and choose to follow through with positive thoughts and actions in ways that are right for you.

Getting back to good will actively enhance your life, but some good, honest effort and planning will need to go into this process. I have listed 10 important steps as general guidelines, but let me emphasize that these steps are placed in no particular order by me, as that can only be done by you. What is important to you can only be decided by, that's right — you. The only thing I will say is that each step is fundamentally important to the process.

10 Steps to Get Back to Good:

1. Have faith.

2. Find a path to goodness that is right for you.

3. Be tolerant and respectful of the countless views and perspectives of goodness that exist.

4. Give thanks every day for all that comes into your life, both good and (seemingly) bad.

5. Accept the fact that you are selfish to a degree by nature, but also acknowledge you maintain excessive selfishness by choice.

6. Look within to change. Identify and reduce selfishness by working to incorporate selfless thoughts and actions into your life.

7. Practice giving. Give help, patience, tolerance, and kindness; give forgiveness, love, and care for others. Give as much as possible; nothing is too big or too small.

8. Nurture all aspects of your health. You must feel good about yourself in order to help others to the best of your ability.

9. Find and fulfill complete purpose for life by caring for your needs as well as the needs of others and nature.

10. Be good. Continually foster as much goodness as possible. There will be times when you may falter, but always work to find your way back to good.

~ Having Faith ~

Many people have faith. In fact, I would venture to say that almost every person on the planet has faith in one way or another. Different perspectives and opinions on this subject have spawned numerous names, concepts, and beliefs reflecting our vast social, cultural and personal differences. These views vary widely and range from having faith in the goodness of humanity to having spiritual faith.

For our purposes here, different views and manners of having faith fit into our collective definition as long as goodness remains a priority. Please use names, concepts, and beliefs regarding faith that you deem appropriate and feel right for you. Having faith, whether spiritually or inherently, is largely a matter of personal belief, opinion, and life experience.

~ Connecting With Goodness ~

Every person owns a unique, personal view, and as such, there are countless ways to establish connections to goodness. The manner in which a person chooses to have faith is an immensely personal choice, and every person knows what feels right on an individual level. Remember, true faith fosters goodness, selflessness, tolerance, care, and compassion, completely rejecting separation, intolerance, causing harm, and narrow-mindedness. Ironically, a major portion of the prejudice, intolerance, and suffering that afflicts our world stems from selfish views of goodness.

Having faith creates many responsibilities. Some of the greatest of those responsibilities are to live with goodness and be tolerant of the various, diverse paths others choose. Different cultures and individuals have unique ways of believing, thinking, and worshipping, just as you may. In the end however, to have faith means very little if it is not followed through with behavior that fosters goodness and tolerance..

~ Giving Thanks ~

The next step in getting back to good is to be thankful for everything in life. I admit that is easier said than done, but a true attitude of gratitude allows an appreciation of the fact that everything in life is a gift, and helps us stop taking things for granted. Many people are not fully aware of what they have received in life, and mere inconveniences or normal challenges somehow grow into problems, while true difficulties unnecessarily turn into disasters.

Unfortunately, when people take things for granted, a sense of entitlement often follows. You may be discouraged with the turns your life has taken and instead of being thankful, perhaps you think, "Why me? Why do I have to suffer or struggle? What did I do to deserve this? It's not fair!"

Completely understanding, noticing, and appreciating the gifts you receive every day can change such perspectives. When you are truly grateful, many 'problems' in life turn out not be problems at all, merely selfish perceptions. Learn to feel blessed for what you have, and remember why you have it. Resolve any sense of entitlement by recognizing all of life's gifts, even the day itself, and remember to *give thanks*.

~ Selfish to Selfless ~

Human beings are selfish by nature. To care for ourselves, our loved ones, and the things we hold dear, we must be selfish to a certain degree — that is a fact of life. The task of caring for that which is important and close to us is natural and normal, but we can mistakenly do it to an excessive degree by excluding and neglecting others. As we care for individual needs, we may become excessively selfish, materialistic, or extreme in aspects of life, while choosing to ignore the fact that others have needs, as well.

Selfishness easily spills over into areas of life where it doesn't belong. By choosing to ignore the fact that others have needs just as important as our own, negativity creates emotions, attitudes, and actions that lead away from goodness. We may become mean, jealous, spiteful, or intolerant of beliefs and physical differences, while encouraging ignorance and hatred.

Getting back to good requires selfish thoughts and actions to be replaced with selflessness. This requires time and effort and often begins with the willingness to admit you are selfish in some ways. Simply because you may have health, money, or success, you should not exist to care solely for that which is important to you. Look beyond self-service and embrace selflessness.

~ Practice Giving ~

A major component of getting back to good is to give selflessly to others. Thoughts and actions are the only things you truly "own" in this life to give. As the keeper of your kindness, your tolerance, your positive attitude of gratitude, and your patience, you have the responsibility to give those things, share them often.

All ways of giving are connected, and each one matters. At heart, they are one and the same. When you give kindness, you are giving help. When you are tolerant, you are being kind. When you are patient and polite, you give help, kindness, and tolerance. There are literally billions of ways to offer goodness, and the extent or amount you are able to give makes no difference; the important thing is *to give*.

The truest sense of giving means to do so because you know in your heart it is the right thing to do, not because you expect to get something in return. Learn to define your purpose as more than caring for you and yours. Choose to reach out and find ways to add value to your life and the lives of others by finding ways to give.

~ Nurture Yourself ~

In order to promote goodness, you must put yourself first — to a certain extent. Having some degree of physical, emotional, and spiritual health is necessary in order to offer goodness to your full potential, because feeling unhealthy affects outlooks and attitudes negatively.

If you notice areas in life that require attention, find effective ways to care for them. While the responsibility to care for yourself is ultimately your own, you don't have to do it alone. Many avenues and resources are available to help improve every aspect of your well-being. Remember, a strong desire to live with goodness is dramatically weakened if you do not choose to take care.

~ Finding Meaning ~

Have you ever felt you are missing something in life or constantly searching for something more? People instinctively search for meaning and purpose, and this need must be satisfied in many different ways in order to feel complete. You can succeed in a career, by raising a family, or accomplishing your goals and dreams, but you may still feel life lacks a complete sense of purpose.

Many of us make the mistake of becoming so involved with the search for purpose that we look right past or through reasons for it. We can lose sight of life's meaning when we become overly focused on our wants, our needs, and our lives. To put it in simple terms: We can find complete purpose for life by achieving our goals and dreams while connecting with, and fostering true goodness.

~ Start Your Journey Now ~

By choosing to maintain a positive perspective, an attitude of gratitude, and a commitment to be a giving person, you will encourage selflessness and experience a genuine, tangible feeling for life. Remember, by getting back to good health and relationships, or in a broader sense, goodness travels through you into our world. Try to engage others with compromise and compassion, while not segregating or alienating the many different ways others choose to express their views. Differing perspectives and characteristics can be beautiful and eye opening, so learn how to include rather than exclude different people, ideas, and beliefs.

Setting Goals:

Goal setting is a powerful process for thinking about what you want to accomplish in your future. Just as important, it motivates you to turn the vision of this future into reality. The process of setting goals helps you know precisely what you want to achieve, and where you'll have to concentrate your efforts and energies.

Goals that are set properly can be incredibly motivating, allowing you quickly spot distractions that may send you in another direction. As you get into the habit of setting and achieving goals to get back to good, you'll find that life will give back to you in untold, positive ways.

Now that you have a basic overview of what getting back to good entails, I want you to set some goals for yourself, and write down why you need to accomplish these goals, which can cover any aspect of your life. You may want to get back to good health by committing to change your lifestyle. Perhaps you will set a goal of being thankful everyday and reflect on your blessings in a gratitude journal. Maybe you will set a goal to take the first step to fix a relationship with someone close to you. These positive intentions will bring you direction and focus on your journey back to good.

As you continue your journey, be sure to make use of the To-Do checklists, note pages, and goal setting lists at the end of the chapters. Also, be sure to capture your thoughts and progress with the journal provided at the back of the book.

MY GOALS TO
GET BACK TO GOOD

Date:_____

- _____
- _____
- _____
- _____
- _____
- _____
- _____
- _____
- _____
- _____
- _____
- _____
- _____
- _____

CHAPTER 3

THE TIE THAT BINDS...
HAVING FAITH

*"Take the first step in faith. You don't have to
see the whole staircase, just take the first step."*
-Dr. Martin Luther King, Jr.

Humanity's vast and varied beliefs have developed into connections to goodness. Throughout history, countless religions and belief systems have formed, changed splintered, and transformed. While much of the compassion, forgiveness, and care exhibited by humanity stems from religious and spiritual beliefs, unfortunately, much of the bloodshed, intolerance, and negativity can be traced to skewed interpretations of spiritual faith due to intolerance. The very teachings of love and compassion among spiritual beliefs that are designed to help us find more goodness and care for one another, have often been distorted and selfishly interpreted to feed a large amount of negativity into our world. This occurred thousands of years ago and continues this very afternoon.

While faith inexorably links to religious and spiritual belief, it is paradoxically solitary on a personal level. My intentions here are not to debate religion and science, or to make a case for particular beliefs, as those subjects can be debated and rationalized by experts and opinionarians. We have more important work to do improving our lives and bringing more goodness in our world.

You have the prerogative to define and interpret faith in your own way. That faith can be in something greater — something more than the here and now. Or, it may be faith in the goodness of humankind and nature. You can even choose to have faith in randomness and happenstance — the choice is yours. Only you know what works and feels right for yourself, but always try to remember that one important aspect of faith is a tolerant connection to goodness.

No matter what names, beliefs, or concepts are associated with faith, it remains a common thread tying humanity together. It binds you to me, and both of us to every person on the planet. It also weaves humanity into the garment of nature — something common to all. Unfortunately, much time and negative energy is spent on pointing out differences of creed, beliefs, and faith. Instead, let's express and experience faith each in our own way, and spend our energy on creative, helpful, healthy pursuits of humanity.

> *"Faith is the strength by which*
> *a shattered world will emerge into the light."*
> **-Helen Keller**

Faith in goodness lends stability and purpose to life, directs you toward a path of righteousness, and exists through your thoughts and actions of gratitude. Your faith something that works for you; but no matter what path you choose, remember that true faith includes thoughts and actions of goodness. While the choice to have faith is one you are free to make, having faith is more than an acknowledgment; it means accepting that giving goodness must be a priority in your life, and taking action to make that a reality.

~Spiritual Connections~

"Thank God. Thank Goodness." Those words are uttered countless times every day around the world because much of humanity maintains spiritual faith. That faith plays such an important role in peoples' lives and is so deep-rooted in the human psyche, that we must take a moment to explore some characteristics of spirituality.

Spiritual faith can be one of the most comforting aspects of our existence, providing support, understanding, and guidance through different situations. In addition, it can bring great joy, peace of mind, and meaning to life. Most importantly, a spiritual connection helps foster goodness toward yourself, your loved ones, those you may not personally know, and to the natural world around you.

Nature is such a miracle that even with our advanced ability to comprehend, its inexplicable complexity and beauty remains considerably beyond our grasp, etching burning questions deep into the human psyche regarding meaning, purpose, and life itself. When reflecting on the magnificence of the natural world around us, and the profound experiences we are capable of, an inherent feeling and knowledge of something greater becomes evident for many people. Albert Einstein eloquently spoke to this matter: "Everyone who is seriously interested in the pursuit of science becomes convinced that a spirit is manifest in the laws of the universe — a spirit vastly superior to man, and one in the face of which our modest powers must feel humble."

All in all, spirituality helps guide us to be thankful, kind, giving, and tolerant. To care for your fellow human beings and nature as you do yourself, and to offer gratitude for all you are given. By choosing to maintain a spiritual connection, you are choosing to accept the responsibility of living with goodness, and remaining tolerant and respectful of differing beliefs. True spiritual teachings do not advocate intolerance or harm.

~ Finding Your Path ~

All connections to goodness, whether personal or of an organized nature, commonly share basic tenets — to act with goodness and humility, to be thankful, selfless, kind, and tolerant (essentially the foundation for the Ethic of Reciprocity or Golden-Rule). Of course, specific views, practices, and sacred doctrines differentiate various beliefs, but differing beliefs can share an equal place in our world when carried out with goodness. Spiritual faith should not cause or encourage intolerance, indifference, or violence, even to the smallest degree.

Every person has a unique spiritual opinion and outlook (even having no belief is a unique spiritual view), and no matter how faith is viewed, I believe we are born with instincts that give us inherent knowledge of goodness. The blueprints for goodness, if you will, are already in place, what you build from those blueprints is up to you.

~ Focus On Goodness and Tolerance ~

*"Religions are many and diverse,
but reason and goodness are one."*

-Elbert Hubbard

People can focus so intensely on material aspects of faith that they neglect to give the appropriate amount of attention to core teachings of goodness. As such, fundamental reasons for faith become obscured. Remember, as important as material aspects and specific practices are to particular beliefs, they are merely tools to help you think about, reflect on, and accomplish connections to goodness. Balance the needs and requirements of your beliefs with thoughts and actions of goodness; concentrate on being thankful, practicing your faith in earnest, acting kindly, and reaching out to others.

Spiritual convictions are often so strong and profound that tolerating and respecting different views can be difficult for some people, leading to the ubiquitous problem of intolerance. When people believe one particular view or way is superior, and try to force those convictions onto others, problems inevitably result. This often sours faith with intolerance and separation, leading away from the goodness that teaches us to become as tolerant as possible in every aspect of life.

Learn to look beyond personal prejudice or bias toward different beliefs and creeds by acknowledging the goodness all faiths and beliefs can share. Ultimately, you choose a connection to goodness that feels right and works for you. Please give others the freedom to do the same. Remember, goodness is a tie that binds, and spiritual interpretations that are laced with intolerance break that binding tie.

Even though much of humanity maintains spiritual beliefs, and countless houses of worship instruct followers to live with goodness, the unfortunate reality is that many of those teachings do not make it out the front door to become thoughts and actions of goodness in the world. Similarly, fundamental instructions of goodness that are the inspired word of many holy texts, read by billions of people of differing beliefs, often do not make it off the written page to become thoughts and actions of goodness. Instead, spiritual beliefs are selfishly incorporated into personal needs, wants, and desires.

Your choice to have faith is free and personal, and the manner in which you make that connection is unique and individual. When choosing to have faith, do your best to think and act with goodness.

"…what matters is that one be a good, kind and warmhearted person. A deep sense of caring for others, based on a profound sense of interconnection, is the essence of the teachings of all great religions of the world."

-The Dalai Lama

✓ To Do List: Connecting With Goodness

❏ **Connect with goodness:**

➢ Choose to accept the responsibility to live with goodness.

➢ Do not cause harm, be intolerant, act selfishly, or foster hatred, *especially* in the name of a spiritual belief.

➢ Negotiate any perceived problems in life with the courage faith provides.

❏ **Realize the purpose of spirituality:**

➢ To connect with goodness.

➢ Focus on being thankful.

➢ Think and act with selflessness.

➢ Have faith.

❏ **If you choose a spiritual connection of faith, focus on the true message of your beliefs:**

➢ Be thankful, practice your faith in earnest, act kindly, and live with tolerance.

➢ Do not focus on material aspects and specific practices of a spiritual belief to the point where you are not promoting goodness.

❏ **Become tolerant of differing spiritual views.**

➢ Understand that different religions, belief systems, and personal views come in many styles, shapes, and sizes, in order to fit the different, dynamic needs and circumstances of humanity.

➤ Illuminate the basic meaning of faith by showing tolerance of differing beliefs.

➤ Learn about and respect different beliefs to avoid spiritual tunnel vision.

My Goals to
Connect with Goodness

Date:_____

- _____
- _____
- _____
- _____
- _____
- _____
- _____
- _____
- _____
- _____
- _____
- _____
- _____
- _____

Notes — Connecting with Goodness:

Notes — Connecting with Goodness:

CHAPTER 4

LOOK UP...
BEING THANKFUL

*"Gratitude is not only the greatest
of virtues, but the parent of all the others."*
—Marcus Tullius Cicero

As I walk out of my apartment each morning, I look at the plaque hung purposefully next to the door; it reads, "Begin Each Day with a Grateful Heart." Thankfulness is a perspective that should encompass every aspect of life. Most of us know saying thank you for what we receive is the right thing to do. We offer thanks to others for holding the door open, for helping us through tough situations, and for giving us gifts. Many times, however, we forget to say thank you or do not feel grateful for what we receive everyday.

A thankful perspective is so powerful that you can find happiness and peace of mind no matter what challenges come your way. Without it, you can become unhappy or despondent with life even if you have a great state of affairs. While feeling grateful when all is going well is relatively easy, as soon as adversity strikes, losing an outlook of gratitude can be just as easy. Try not to complain, feel mad, or become sad when facing challenging situations. Granted, this may be difficult to do and will take time to learn how to put into action, but doing so will allow you to better tolerate adversity. Try to find something to be grateful for every day.

~ The Foundation of Thankfulness ~

In order for you to achieve an attitude of gratitude, strengthen views that support your foundation of thankfulness and remove obstacles that chip and rot that foundation away. No one can force you to feel grateful or make you see the goodness and positive things that exist in your life. That point of view must come from you.

- **Remember and strengthen these views:**
    1. Simply be thankful.
    2. Be grateful for each new day.
    3. Be thankful for your health.
    4. Be thankful for your abilities.
- **Remove these obstacles:**
    1. Taking things for granted.
    2. Feeling entitled.
    3. Dealing with tough, tragic times without a thankful perspective.
    4. Pitying yourself because of your problems.
    5. Worrying about situations you have no control over.
- **Maintain your thankful perspective:**
    1. Your thankful checklist / gratitude journal.
    2. That's life!
    3. Thankfulness can be achieved.

~ **Strengthen Your Thankful Perspective** ~

Although it may not be possible to feel genuinely grateful all the time, wholeheartedly putting these insights into practice will help you feel thankful more often without giving it a second thought.

1: Simply Be Thankful.

Feeling grateful for everything in life leads to a life without overwhelming problems, struggles, or hardship. This is not to say you won't experience tough, troubling, or challenging situations, because everyone does; however, feeling genuinely thankful gives you a positive perspective that can combat the negative effects of adversity and allow you to focus on being grateful for the big picture.

Try to be mindful of the fact that everything in life is given to you — even the day itself. Sure, you may own things on paper or have your name associated with achievements, titles, or positions, but ultimately you only have such things because they have been given to you. Show gratitude every day with your thoughts *and* through your actions.

2: Be Grateful For Each New Day

While it is important to feel thankful for waking each day, and for what is in your life, it is also necessary to remember that humankind collectively receives a gift with every new sunrise. The possibility exists that some type of celestial or natural event, such as a meteor impact, a super-volcanic eruption, or other catastrophic disaster could befall our planet and totally annihilate life as we know it. Granted, the odds of such an event are extremely small, but the possibility does exist. And there is always the more realistic possibility of the hundreds of different, "smaller" natural disasters that could throw our lives into chaos at any time around the neighborhood or around the world. These scenarios are not written to scare or proclaim 'the end is near,' but to help you remember how small humanity is in the overall scheme of existence.

We have invented, discovered, and created many magnificent things, but they pale in comparison to the natural world. Our technological advancements and discoveries are insignificant when contrasted by forces of nature, and overconfidence in our abilities can lead us to forget our power is as fragile and feeble as life itself. Any human progress and achievement relies on the fact that we are given each new day, as our advancements would not be possible without the opportunities nature affords us.

Life exists on this planet only as long as the sun continues to shine and rain continues to fall. Be grateful for each new day by acknowledging every day as a gift that should not be taken for granted. Be humble and show thanks for the awesome power and splendor of nature by treating it with respect.

The Essence of a New Day

This is the beginning of a new day. You have been given this day to use as you will. You can waste it or use it for good. What you do today is important because you are exchanging a day of your life for it. When tomorrow comes, this day will be gone forever; in its place is something that you have left behind…let it be something good.

—Author Unknown

3: Be Thankful For Your Health

Once you have offered thanks for the dawning of each new day, be thankful for the health you have. The first step in doing so is recognizing that health is not yours; it is a gift. Of course, you have the responsibility to care for yourself, but even if you work hard to maintain a healthy lifestyle, you can become afflicted with disease and disability. When blessed with health in any aspect, be thankful, and use it to bring more goodness into your life.

Everything in nature is designed to have a limited existence, from the six hundred year old redwood tree to the three-day life of a mosquito. Be mindful of the fact that age happens and illness occurs. Try not to feel mad, sad, or cheated when health problems confront you, as aging and illness are a natural part of life, and only become an unmanageable issue when self-pity takes over. Self-pity rears its head when we start asking, "Why me? Why do I have to suffer?" In truth, the question we should be asking is, "Why not me?" Always remember to be thankful every day for health because it can be gone in an instant!

4: Be Thankful For your Abilities

We often neglect to be thankful in recognizing our natural abilities. In order to achieve, you may have to sacrifice, toil through difficult situations, and work diligently to accomplish your goals; giving you a feeling of pride and a sense of satisfaction. Those feelings are normal and healthy up to a certain point. While you must put forth the effort, sacrifice, and work for your achievements, the only reason you are able to accomplish them is because you are *given* you what you need to do so (i.e. the day itself, health, talents, etc).

An overabundance of pride in your abilities or achievements shows an ignorance of gratitude, which can cause you to believe you are better than other people. When you feel superior, you are not acting in a thankful manner. Do you know people who treat others poorly because of differing degrees of material possessions, abilities, status, or achievements? If you recognize these behaviors in yourself, immediately take thankful action by grounding yourself to the fact that you are given what you need in order to achieve what you attain. Remember, you are equal to everyone no matter your status or pursuits in life.

Maintaining a thankful perspective means feeling blessed to be as smart, creative, and successful as you are. When you view abilities as gifts, you will not feel superior, and will treat others equally — with respect, no matter how accomplishments, status, educational level, or social group differs from your own.

~ Removing Obstacles ~

Reducing obstacles that hinder an attitude of gratitude is the next necessary step to a thankful perspective. Learn to recognize when and where these obstacles appear in your life and work to remove them.

1: Taking For Granted

Stop taking things for granted. That phrase is very clichéd — only because it is so very correct! People can be self-centered, taking many aspects of life for granted. Overlooking the fact that everything you have, no matter how large or small, is a gift can be easy. All too often, life is turned upside down in the blink of an eye by hardship or tragedy, and unfortunately, this is often the only time many people realize their blessings. Another cliché testifies to that fact: "You don't know what you've got until it's gone." The wisdom of these clichés is not to be ignored. You can agree with them now or be forced to accept them later.

In order to become more thankful, start with the simple act of noticing what you have in front of you every day. Make a list of all you are grateful for and establish a daily routine to reflect on these gifts. Remember what you have — from your health, to your loved ones, to another day — and you will begin to achieve a more thankful attitude by *choosing* to take nothing for granted.

2: I'm Entitled To That!

When you take life for granted, a sense of entitlement frequently follows. You may believe you are owed a nice, healthy, prosperous, and rewarding life, but try to view health, happiness, and life as the gifts they are, and be grateful for them.

Do you ever feel entitled rather than thankful? Have you reflected on the fact that the ability to live, achieve, and be successful is a gift? While you may achieve your goals, remember, you are allowed to do these things — not entitled to them. All of your accomplishments and abilities are not entirely your own, and they can be taken from you in an instant. While feeling proud and pleased about achievements and abilities is good, always remain thankful for the fact that you are given the ability to accomplish, and transform any sense of entitlement into thankful actions of goodness.

3: Tough Times — Tragic Times

Terrifying stories or occurrences of hardship, injury, tragedy, and death have touched every one of us in some way. We hear about them on the news, from people we know, or find out firsthand through personal experience. When tragedy strikes, it can be shocking and horrifying. Unfortunately, this is often the only time our eyes are truly open to the reality of what belongs to us — *nothing*. No amount of money or perceived power can undo a tragic accident or death, control nature, or stop undesirable things from happening, as these things are beyond our control.

During tough and tragic times, a selfish, thankless attitude causes you to feel slighted and treated unfairly. In turn, these feelings fuel a host of negative emotions and thoughts. I have often heard people exclaim, "How could this to happen? I've been a good person. Why is this happening to me? It's not fair." When you find yourself asking these questions, you are not thinking as thankfully as possible. Coping with challenges and troubles by remembering all you should be grateful for can keep your perspective in a more positive light.

~ Conquer Difficult Situations ~

Tough, tragic times can be very difficult to cope with, and emotions help you deal with the pain, confusion, and anger you may feel. These feelings are a normal part of the process of learning to cope. However, you can also purposefully apply positive thoughts and actions to encourage a thankful attitude that will lessen the severity and duration of any pain and suffering you may endure.

Coping method 1: *Trust your faith.*

Even if you don't understand why bad things happen, placing trust in your faith with an attitude of gratitude will help replace pain with understanding. How many times has something happened to you that seemed bad, only to turn out to be good in the end? Another cliché comes to mind: "a blessing in disguise."

Sometimes you may feel like there are no answers to your questions. Perhaps you will learn the reason for dire life events or hardships later in life, or even after life. Above all, learn to put faith and trust in your connection to goodness.

Coping method 2: *Accept the fact that adversity is a fact of life.*

Adversity strikes during the course of every lifetime. Loved ones are lost; family members, friends, and innocent people experience tragedy every day. Debilitating illnesses grab hold of people, forcefully squeezing and choking the life out of them. Forces of nature create havoc, tragic accidents occur, and chasms created by humankind seize life, health, and happiness.

How can anyone effectively cope with such things? One way to deal with adversity is to accept it as a natural part of life, in that difficulty and hardship will not always find someone else or happen to the "other person." When adversity appears, find a way to effectively cope with it, and try to understand what you need to learn from it. Although finding gratitude in some situations may seem impossible, confront adversity with the strength and positive attitude a thankful perspective provides.

Coping method 3: *Think of how any given situation could be worse.*

Try not to get caught up in the "Why me?" syndrome, which combines discouragement with self-pity. When facing tough times or hardship, you may feel horrible, helpless, and angry. STOP! Granted, these emotions and feelings are part of a process to help you cope, but try to be thankful your circumstances are only as bad as they are, because every situation could be worse. When dealing with adversity, you may not be able to change your situation, but you can change your perspective.

- *Here are two tips to help you cope with tough times and situations:*

First, visualize completely unbearable circumstances. For example, if a loved one has suffered traumatic injuries in a terrible accident, you will undoubtedly be scared, worried, and feel terrible about seeing her in such a situation. However, imagine you lost your loved one in that accident. Think and reflect upon what that would be like. Dream in vivid detail about the memorial service, the lonely holidays, and the emptiness in your home. Jump back to reality and be thankful for what you do have — your situation is not as bad as it could be. Another example; perhaps you just found out that a loved one has cancer; bad news to say the least. However, instead of lamenting the fact that this bad news has reared its ugly head, try to see your blessings. Sometimes people find out that a loved one has cancer along with having cancer themselves, losing a job, becoming disabled in an accident…the list can go on and on. Almost every situation could be worse.

*When you can't imagine something worse…*Sometimes people face circumstances where they understandably cannot imagine anything worse. At this point, you must turn to faith. Remember, truly connecting to goodness means having faith in *every* situation that crosses your path — not only during the good times.

When enduring the loss of a loved one, remember to be grateful for what you have had with them. Remember the touch, the time, the smiles, and the love. Do not forget those things. At the very least, feel thankful and blessed for the time you were given with him or her.

- *The second tip to help you cope is by remembering a time in your life when you were truly blessed — or downright lucky!*

Let me give you one example from my life. Back when I was living at home with my folks in the late nineties I worked the afternoon shift at the phone company. My parents worked early in the morning and didn't get home until five, so every day I would let our dogs out in the yard before I left. The day in question started out like every other day. I woke up, said good-by to my parents as they left for work and went about my morning routine. I worked out, showered, wasted time in front of the tv and computer, and let the dogs out.

Around eleven it was time to go. But being the chronic procrastinator that I am, I waited until eleven thirty. Of course, by this time I was in a mad rush to get out the door. I ran to my truck in the driveway and started it up. Now keep in mind that my truck was a twenty-two foot long, four-door pickup with a manual transmission, and our driveway was uphill from the road. As the truck warmed up, I remembered thinking "Did I let the dogs in?" I couldn't remember, so out the truck I went, running to the back yard.

Sure enough, my two black labs, Pepper and Jack sat there wagging their tails at me from the other side of the fence. I hurriedly hopped the fence and let them in the house. I knew I was going to be late for work, so I darted back around the house to my driveway. As I rounded the garage, my truck was gone! A thought instantly raced through my head — someone saw it running and drove it ... but before I could even finish my thought I noticed the truck just sitting in the middle of my street, blocking traffic. "Oh ----," I thought to myself, I didn't set the parking brake

Now, my street wasn't the busiest street in the world, but there was a fair amount of traffic, and cars were stopped in the road on both sides of my truck. I remember fearing the worst and thinking, "The big Ford rolled down the driveway uncontrollably and hit a poor kid on a bike, or a mom walking her baby, or the elderly gentleman that made his daily trek around the block. Oh man, did I screw up!"

I ran down to the street, anxious and embarrassed, and when I got to the front of my pick up, I timidly walked to the back to see what I had done. I saw some reddish fluid around the back tire, and my heart nearly stopped. Peering around the bumper simultaneously answered my prayers and calmed my fears. The back axle had bumped into a small boulder in my neighbor's yard and dented the shock absorber, which was now leaking.

Thankfully, no one was injured (or worse) and there was no damage to anything except my brakes, unless you count my ego. I solemnly climbed into the driver's seat and pulled back up the driveway to let the other vehicles by.

Call this situation what you will: fate, luck, coincidence, or an angel on my shoulder. No matter what you call it or how you view it, this was and always will be a situation for which I will be thankful. I am grateful that my life did not change that day in ways it certainly could have. And I choose to remember the gift I was given that day, during good times in my life and especially during the rough patches.

When you are facing adversity, think about the days and situations you have to be grateful for — each one of us has at least one and likely many more. Take some time to reflect on those 'lucky days' in your life, write them down, and feel grateful. Change your perspective to an attitude of gratitude, and you will deal with adversity in a much more positive way.

Coping method 4: *Dealing with adversity gets easier as time passes.*

To understand this coping method, it is necessary to look back at some occasion when you were in a great deal of physical pain. Perhaps you suffered an injury or had an operation. At the time, the pain may have felt unbearable, but somehow you managed to get through it. Can you recall feeling the pain to the same degree and intensity that you felt while actually going through the situation? Probably not. Of course, you may remember the ordeal as being painful, but the point to understand here is that it no longer affects you in the same way — it does not hurt to the same degree.

Suffering from physical pain is similar to experiencing tragedy, hardship, or loss. The first days, months, and even years can seem unbearable. However, with time and a thankful outlook, the pain will subside. Remember to view life in the biggest possible picture and maintain trusting faith. When all is said and done, every experience you have will be a memory, leaving only your outlook. Make that outlook a positive, thankful one, and tough, trying, or tragic times can no longer affect you in the same way.

4: Self-Pity

If you forget that adversity makes you stronger, it's all too easy to wallow in self-pity instead of giving thanks. You may have worrisome problems and troubles, but try not to think your situation is the most challenging, tough, or grim circumstance anyone has ever handled. By pitying yourself and your circumstances, you are not being thankful for what you have.

At times, life can certainly be difficult; there is no question about that. Many people think they have grave problems, but the fact of the matter is most of us do not. When we compare our problems to some of the real tragedies in our world, we soon realize our troubles are often a by-product of a selfish perspective.

I have come to know an older couple that provides a good example of feeling pity instead of thankfulness. They were healthy all their lives, worked hard, and earned a good living that provided enough money to purchase a nice house, put food on the table, and still have some money in the bank. However, as sickness and general old age set in, they seemed to forget their many, many blessings.

In the process of dealing with their present situation, they chose to see only the immediate problems and pain that confronted them, and forgot about their blessings of health, prosperity and a healthy, happy family. They failed to maintain a thankful view by not recognizing the absolute bounty they had received over the years.

If this couple were to look back on their lives with an attitude of gratitude, they would feel blessed for being healthy for a majority of life, as well as for their healthy family. Sure, the pain would still exist, and age would still take its toll; however, they would realize just how much they had received. A perspective of thankfulness would allow them to better cope with their current situation and empathize with the struggles other people go through, instead of becoming increasingly withdrawn, jealous, and embittered because of self-pity.

Thankful perspective: Try not to pity yourself because of your circumstances; be happy your situation is not worse. If you are going through a tough time, do not compare your pain and suffering to the blessings others may be receiving. Be thankful for your life, empathetic to the trials people go through, and happy for others when good fortune embraces them.

Everyone will face tough times at some point, and feeling slighted seems normal *only if* you do not have a thankful perspective. In fact, it is indeed easy for most people to pity themselves when they are selfishly preoccupied with what they think belongs to them. Self-pity is a negative characteristic that can be erased with a perspective of gratitude.

5: Worry, Worry, Go Away...Relax!

Another major obstacle to being thankful is the very human need to feel in control of life. People can be overcome with worry and speculation very easily when they don't realize just how much is out of the realm of personal control. While there are variables and situations that can be managed, such as how hard you work, how much effort you put into life, and the choices you make, ultimately you control very little. How many times do people plan for a certain outcome and everything goes awry? Situations and circumstances are often out of our hands, and we can fail to remember or recognize that fact.

> *"Never let the future disturb you.*
> *You will meet it, if you have to,*
> *with the same weapons of reason*
> *which today arm you against the present."*
> **-Marcus Aurelius**

Concern and care (a.k.a. worry) have a place and purpose, but excessive or misplaced worrying brings about negative thoughts and perspectives. This negativity spreads into all aspects of life and affects everything from your health to your interaction with others. For instance, I was involved with a wedding that was planned out meticulously. Every detail was planned, re-planned, and then thought about some more. The soon-to-be newlyweds were trying the patience and kindness of everyone who was helping them prepare for the big event, because they were getting a little obsessive about the whole production.

The young couple would not stand for something going wrong with the wedding. By focusing narrowly on their particular wants and wishes, they became unnecessarily anxious and angry toward each other and their family and friends. They generated feelings of nervousness, stress, and anger because they wanted complete control. Those feelings negatively affected everything about the situation.

Following months and months of planning, the big day arrived. After extracting every bit of energy and goodwill from themselves and those around them, the bride and groom were set. A few hours before the wedding was to start, the groom's father went on a last-minute errand. As the clock ticked closer to the wedding hour, he had not returned and everyone started to get understandably anxious. The time for the ceremony to start passed...fifteen minutes...forty minutes...an hour went by. Regrettably, the wedding party received the unwelcome news that the groom's father had suffered a massive heart attack and was in intensive care at a local hospital.

Thankful perspective: Try not to become so involved with trying to control life that you forget what is important. Losing sight of what you really control and becoming too involved with the details of life is a recipe for a rude awakening. Adversity finds everyone at some point and in some way — that is a fact over which you have no control. Do not entertain the notion that it will not find you. Granted, a wedding can be a most stressful time, and this particular wedding scenario may be an extreme example, but try to keep your sense of control in check regarding details and situations in life.

***

We can prepare for situations within our control, and plan for the future responsibly and carefully; but worrying about what is beyond our control causes unnecessary stress and obscures a thankful perspective.

***

Learn to let go of the uncontrollable aspects of life and pour that energy into being grateful in thought, attitude, and action. Most of us are blessed at one time or another. Remember those times and be thankful for them. When you feel worried — try to Stop! Give thanks for what you do have.

~ Maintain a Thankful Perspective ~

As you incorporate thankfulness into your life and remove obstacles that hinder it, you can actively practice methods to help it take root and remain strong. Remember, your perception of life can allow you to find peace of mind and fulfillment regardless of what comes your way.

1: Your Thankful Checklist

The everyday things in life are so important that you should be thankful for them as often as you can. I recognize that it is impossible to feel thankful 100 percent of the time, and everyone is guilty of taking things for granted, but establishing and reflecting on a "I am Thankful For" checklist / gratitude journal can help you strengthen your thankful perspective. Simply make a checklist of all you are grateful for in life. Keep a copy close to your hand as well as your heart. Inventory the contents of your list frequently and constantly find more to add to it. Make it a habit to review your list daily.

First, be thankful for waking. Feel blessed to have another day — not just a day for you and your loved ones, but be grateful that the world has another sunrise. Now, if you can feel, give thanks. Can you hear? Can you see? Can you move at all? Can you think with a clear mind? If you answered yes to just one of these questions, be thankful. If you can say yes to more than one, consider yourself truly blessed.

Be grateful every day for your health. If you are not healthy in some aspect, you can be thankful for the times you were healthy and for your current health in other areas. The same goes for your loved ones. Are your loved ones well now or have they had health at one time? Do not forget these times simply because they may be gone — give thanks for them.

Review your list often and let thoughts of thankfulness permeate your mind. Over time, they will serve to strengthen an attitude of gratitude and work magic with your perspective. Continually add more items to your "Things To Be Thankful For" checklist and remember to review it daily. Give thanks for all that is in your life by consciously recognizing what you have been given.

2: That's Life

Challenging circumstances and down right awful things can happen to anyone at any time. Life can be turned upside-down and changed forever in an instant. The difficulties of life fall upon everyone. One person may enjoy life at a particular moment while another may be suffering through tragedy. Everyone goes through trials, tribulations, and moments of negativity, but what determines success in dealing with adversity is the strength of your attitude of gratitude.

Accept the fact that life may not turn out exactly as you desire. A key factor in remaining forever thankful is to accept that adversity will strike in some way, so don't be surprised when adversity comes to rest on you — it won't always happen to someone else. So many times I've heard people say, "I never thought this could happen to me." Make every effort to remain consciously aware of the fact that something like "that" could happen to you at any time. Of course you shouldn't spend time worrying about the many bad things that could happen, but be willing to accept the fact that you are not immune from difficulties or tough, tragic times.

All too often, we don't realize what we have until strong adversity is bearing down on us. If you are facing real tragedy, try to remember what life was like before you were presented with serious problems. Do you look at others who are complaining about trivial or petty problems and tell yourself, "If I only had your problems?" Learn to view petty problems and inconveniences as what they truly are by remembering life could always be worse.

Life can seem rough and unfair, but as my grandmother always told me, "The sun can't shine every day." There is much wisdom in that statement. Clouds and rain are just as important to our lives as the sun. Similarly, we need troubling times in life so we can learn from them, grow from them, and appreciate our good times more because of them. Difficult times ultimately prove to be as necessary to life as the good ones.

Life can be hard, but life happens. Cope with it while being thankful and fostering goodness. Do not be afraid of adversity, and try not to complain too much. That's life — give thanks for it.

3: Thankfulness Can Be Achieved!

If it seems impossible to maintain an attitude of gratitude in your situation, remember that many people are able to do so during the most dire and dark circumstances imaginable. Interestingly, those who maintain a thankful perspective when tragedy strikes stand out like a lighthouse to a ship that is miles from shore.

At a funeral of a child, a grieving single father was obviously distressed and sad, but he was the first to point out he was thankful for the time he was given with his child. He did not pity himself because he lost his wife in a car accident a year earlier, and he did not pity himself through this very tough ordeal. He was grieving, of course, but he stayed focused on the fact that nothing in life was truly his, and maintained strong faith. This perspective helped him remain thankful throughout his ordeal.

Another incident of a truly thankful perspective is demonstrated by the following event. A family was driving on an expressway with Mom, Dad, and four children in the car. In the blink of an eye, a horrible accident caused an explosion to tear through the back of the vehicle. All four children perished in the flames. Amazingly, the parents, although distraught, were still able to be thankful for their children. They were hurt and grieving, but they were able to trust in something greater than the here and now.

The third example of thankfulness brings us to a town that had just been ravaged by a tornado. A local news crew was interviewing area residents. One newscaster approached a woman who was in hysterics. Her husband and child were standing next to her as she cried about losing everything.

"How could this happen?" she cried. "This is why we moved to this part of the country! Now we have nothing! Nothing!" Fortunately, she did not lose her family and no loved ones were hurt, but she was having trouble seeing the good in that news.

The newscaster moved to another woman across the street. Her family was safe, and she had lost all of her possessions in the storm, as well. However, this woman held a strong perspective of thanks.

The first words she spoke were, "Thank God my family is okay. It is only by the grace of God that we are still here. I know many other people are not so lucky, and my heart goes out to them."

The difference a thankful perspective can make is astounding. Two different people suffered similar losses, yet one perceives she has lost everything, while another believes she has been given everything.

A final example of positive thankfulness comes from some of my best friends, Dawn and Gary. They are a married couple who bring warmth, friendliness and positive energy wherever they go by putting the needs of others first. There came a day when Dawn and Gary had to put themselves first, but not for a selfish reason — Gary was diagnosed with cancer. That news would be enough to knock the wind out of anyone's sails, but despair was not an option for this couple.

Even though they had a two-year-old son, and infant twin boys, Dawn and Gary faced this challenge head on with resounding faith, a thankful perspective, and an unshakable, positive attitude. Smiles never ceased, laughter could still be heard, and their overwhelmingly positive character served to lift not only their spirits, but the spirits of those around them as well. The positive energy of their attitude worked wonders in all directions.

Fortunately, as of this writing, Gary and his family are winning the fight against the scourge of cancer. They know many trials are ahead, but their trusting faith and positive perspective of thankfulness remain unwavering. Ultimately, those things will help them get through any tough and trying times. I admire and respect their strength beyond words and look to the example they set by their actions and attitude as the thankfulness benchmark each of us should aspire to reach.

We all know of situations that are incredibly trying, because millions of examples of tragedy exist. Along with those tragedies and the tough times that go with them are positive examples of people maintaining thankful attitudes. Naturally, it isn't easy to feel thankful in extremely painful situations of tragedy and loss. However, follow the examples of gratitude that people set through adverse situations because it can be done. You can do it, too!

~ Give Thanks ~

Life is a learning process. We can choose to learn from every experience or we can wallow in pity and be thankless when life does not turn out as we plan. At times there is much pain in life, both perceived and real, but we must keep the faith. Always feel a sense of gratitude for the past and present, no matter what comes along.

As your attitude of gratitude becomes stronger, you will learn to accept the fact that nothing is truly yours — every part of life is just a loan, a lease that can be rescinded at any time. When you achieve this perspective, you no longer feel you can lose anything when faced with adversity and hardship, allowing peace of mind.

Even though life can be painful, even unbearable at times, we have to remember that we will eventually understand if we have faith. When people ask why bad things to happen, or why senseless violence occurs in our world every day, remember that we are not privy to understanding the biggest picture. A true perspective of thankfulness allows you to trust your faith for all that happens in life. At the same time, your thankful attitude will give you strength and courage. Care for your needs, plan for the future, and live your life, but always maintain attitudes of gratitude because they help you recognize your gifts.

When life is clouded with selfishness, you cannot maintain a thankful perspective. If you have been blessed with health, opportunities, and the ability to accomplish, remember to *give* thanks. You can *give* thanks by becoming a person who shows gratitude by giving to others. Give money, time, or service. Remember, those things are not yours in the first place — they are gifts to you. Do not be greedy with what you have and give while you are able. Learn to become a selfless, giving person. *Give* thanks.

✓ To Do List: Look Up — Be Thankful

❑ **Be thankful for each new day:**
  ➢ Remember that every day is a gift — for you personally, as well as for the world.

❑ **Are there some tragedies or hardships that you have undergone and become stronger?**
  ➢ Use your experience as a foundation for helping someone else going through a similar challenge.

❑ **Be thankful for your health:**
  ➢ Remember that health is ultimately not in your hands.

❑ **Be thankful for your abilities:**
  ➢ Realize your abilities are gifts.
  ➢ Be humble as you remember accomplishments are not completely yours.

❑ **Remove obstacles that hinder a thankful perspective.**

❑ **Stop taking things for granted:**
  ➢ Consciously think about and be grateful for what is in your life every day.
  ➢ Show gratitude in thought as well as action.

- ➤ Recognize that you are not entitled to health, happiness, or a good life—they are gifts.
- ➤ Be thankful for, and humbled by the gifts you receive.

❏ **Be willing to accept that adversity may strike at any time in life.**

❏ **Be thankful through tough times.**
- ➤ Always find something to be thankful for, no matter what situation you are going through.
- ➤ Find thankful ways to deal with tough situations.

❏ **Do not pity yourself because of circumstances in life:**
- ➤ View life with thankfulness instead of pity.
- ➤ Do not compare your problems with the problems of others.
- ➤ Remember, your situation could always be worse.
- ➤ View adversity as something that will make you stronger.
- ➤ Be happy for others when good fortune embraces them.

❏ **Try not to worry about what cannot be controlled:**
- ➤ Much of life is beyond your control.

➢ Do not get so caught up with the details of life that you forget to act with thankfulness and goodness.

➢ Convert the energy spent on worrying into thankful thoughts and actions.

❏ **Strengthen your thankful perspective.**

❏ **Create your "I am Thankful For:" checklist:**
➢ Reflect on and write down everything you should be thankful for, from a new day, to health, to the goodness of humanity.

➢ Review your checklist several times a day and add to it often.

➢ Establish a routine for daily gratitude.

❏ **Maintain an attitude of gratitude to the best of your ability:**
➢ Take heart in the fact that people have gone through terrible situations and have been able to maintain a thankful perspective. So can you!

➢ Share some of the gifts you receive with others.

➢ Remember that a life clouded with selfishness cannot maintain a thankful perspective.

❏ **Couple your thankful perspective with thankful actions of goodness.**
• Recommended Reading:
  ▪ *The Gratitude Journal* **by Jack Canfield**

I AM THANKFUL FOR:

1. _____
2. _____
3. _____
4. _____
5. _____
6. _____
7. _____
8. _____
9. _____
10. _____
11. _____
12. _____
13. _____
14. _____
15. _____
16. _____
17. _____
18. _____
19. _____
20. _____
21. _____
22. _____
23. _____
24. _____
25. _____
26. _____

I AM THANKFUL FOR:

27. _____
28. _____
29. _____
30. _____
31. _____
32. _____
33. _____
34. _____
35. _____
36. _____
37. _____
38. _____
39. _____
40. _____
41. _____
42. _____
43. _____
44. _____
45. _____
46. _____
47. _____
48. Please add more to this list.

MY GOALS
FOR GRATITUDE

Date:_____

- _____
- _____
- _____
- _____
- _____
- _____
- _____
- _____
- _____
- _____
- _____
- _____
- _____
- _____

Notes — Being Thankful:

Notes — Being Thankful:

CHAPTER 5

LOOK WITHIN TO CHANGE

*"We must look within ourselves to
find that which we seek in others."*

—Ken William

People can find it quite challenging to distinguish the difference between what is genuinely good and what is good for selfish needs and desires. Although an innate knowledge of goodness exists within every person, the reality is that many of us struggle to connect with that knowledge. Personal views and opinions easily become self-serving and conditional, and by selfishly caring for our physical, spiritual, material, and emotional needs, we can forget or even intentionally ignore the fact that other people require fulfillment of their own.

In today's world, perhaps more than ever, selfishness, ignorance, and intolerance can cause us to believe our own experience of life, such as a certain spiritual belief, racial or social group, nationality, or culture is superior. Any differences, no matter how innocent or benign, can become objects of intolerance. If we choose to ignore the fact that we are equally connected, we will continue on a downward spiral of negativity and selfishness.

The problem runs the gamut from countries waging war to people committing crimes and violence to the smaller, selfish interactions of people on an individual basis. Even something as seemingly insignificant as cutting in front of someone in line, giving a rude gesture while driving, or making fun of someone detracts from goodness in the same way, although not to the same degree, as more selfish, violent, or immoral actions.

Though many of us are taught to be selfless by parents, mentors, and religious / spiritual teachings, we often think and behave more selfishly than we should. While some degree of selfishness is necessary for survival, it can be taken beyond that original, positive intent; ranging from having petty arguments or difficulties with those around us, to phenomenal amounts of greed, jealousy, violence, and self-centeredness.

You have the ability to choose to be the working definition of positive or negative, to live with selflessness or to be excessively selfish. Being overly selfish is a *choice* that brings intolerance, greed, and jealousy into our lives. On the other hand, choosing to be selfless by giving to others and fostering kindness, tolerance, and goodness brings you phenomenal amounts of happiness and peace.

~ Why are We Selfish? ~

Selfishness is necessary for survival — a mechanism for self-preservation. In the natural scheme of life, individuals of every species are bound by the innate knowledge of what must be done to survive physically (selfish behaviors). Survival of the fittest is a law of nature stating that the strong will survive. The strong are able to harness what they need through their attributes, talents, and physical abilities, thereby prospering while the weak and less fortunate become a part of history. Nature, outside of humanity, runs perfectly with this design in place because life takes only what it needs. There are no drives or desires other than those for basic survival, with no waste, no want, and no excess.

The self-preservation (selfish) programming that works so well in nature becomes radically changed when applied to human intellect, traits, and emotions. Human beings think and act selfishly because those feelings and tendencies are instinctively wired into the psyche to allow for physical self-preservation; however, problems occur because we can easily incorporate selfishness into areas of life where it does not belong.

~ Why are we Selfless? ~

Survival instincts for human beings are similar to those of other forms of life in many respects, yet have one major difference. While we must maintain life-sustaining behaviors, self-preservation for human beings goes beyond mere physical survival. We seek purpose and meaning for life, which can be fulfilled in large part through selfless instincts.

Why are people selfless when it is not necessary for physical survival? The answer to that question lies in the fact that selflessness fulfills the more complex areas of self-preservation — soul or spirit preservation, if you will. When you give to someone or promote goodness in some way, you are doing something that directly benefits you.

~Our Instincts~

Selfishness is ingrained in the human mind as an instinct, and so is selflessness, but either may seem more or less prevalent in any one person. Verification of the instinctual programming of the human mind is evident in many ways. One such verification is the fact that you feel satisfied when you complete a task related to an instinct. When you are hungry and fulfill that hunger by eating, you feel a sense of satisfaction. When you are thirsty, and drink, you feel good — satisfied. Caring for your needs also brings instinctual fulfillment. Accordingly, we can see selflessness programmed into the mind because when we carry out selfless actions, we feel good. Giving to someone or helping in some way brings a sense of satisfaction that comes from fulfilling selfless instincts.

Another method of determining human instincts is to look at the actions of very young children (approximately 1–2 years old), because human nature is pure and easy to view in the behaviors of young children. The following examples are admittedly elementary, but effectively demonstrate basic instinctual behaviors.

The fact that young children act selfishly is not a new discovery. In fact, they show selfishness in a number of different ways. For instance, if a child wants something and cannot get it, he may cry or throw tantrums until the matter is forgotten or until the desire is satisfied. Another example of selfish behavior occurs when a child has something she is not willing to share. How many parents remember their child saying the words "no!" or "mine!"? If the child has not yet developed speech, she may rely on a piercing scream or slight demonstrations of physical force to communicate the desire to keep what she wants. Is the child consciously thinking about acting in such ways? Has the child been taught to be selfish at this tender age? Of course not. The child simply knows he or she wants something, and the thoughts and actions of pure, selfish instincts are revealed.

Thankfully, children also show actions that are selfless in nature. They may show signs of selfless giving, such as sharing a toy, offering some of their lunch, or maybe even leaving a favorite toy to show compassion and empathy to someone who is hurt. Again, they do not act this way because they are taught to or are consciously thinking about doing so; they inherently know *how* to act selflessly. Such actions are the pure instinctual programming of the human mind translated directly into action.

As children grow, behaviors are molded by experience, rules, instruction, and guidance received from those around them. The upbringing and environment in which a child grows up exerts major influences on perceptions and perspectives that meld with unique traits to form a distinctive personality. These factors work collectively with intellect and emotion to affect the choices and decisions each of us make throughout life.

Selfless instincts must be nurtured and reinforced during formative years in order for them to take root and become a driving force later in life. A person's childhood can be filled with so much negativity that connecting with selfless instincts becomes virtually impossible. Consequently, we must constantly stress the importance of caring for children with love and goodness. While childhood environment plays a major role in the way a person thinks and acts as an adult, we must not use it as an excuse; ultimately, every person is responsible to direct his or her energies toward selfless thoughts and actions.

~ We Choose Our Choices ~

Each of us faces a dilemma as we try to maintain a proper balance between our instincts. How do we balance these driving forces? To a certain extent, our intellect allows us to control instincts with reason, logic, and emotion, although there are times when a person can act or react purely on instinct. The task of controlling or balancing instincts is helped by the innate ability to fundamentally know right from wrong; what we call conscience. Because we are free to choose thoughts and actions, we have the power to interpret and control our instincts, often causing a dilemma for us; selfishness can dominate our selfless intuition quite easily and cause us to think and act more selfishly than we should.

Instincts, personality, and upbringing can only affect us to a certain degree, as we ultimately control and are accountable for thoughts and actions. For instance, if a person has been raised in a selfless home full of goodness, he or she may choose to act selfishly. In contrast, a child who faces a preponderance of selfishness can still grow to become a positive, selfless person.

These outcomes may be a result of external influences, innate behaviors, or a combination of several factors, but they are ultimately the result of choice.

The common urge to blame someone or something else for our behaviors may seem justified at times, but is almost always wrong. Every day we are faced with the task of making decisions, and those decisions can move us toward goodness or cause us to stray from it. At the end of the day, we have the ability to choose our choices.

~ Selfishness is Abundant ~

Although countless thoughts and actions of selflessness occur every day, their effects are diminished by numerous selfish actions. Violent, vicious, and evil actions often capture the spotlight; but selfishness is not limited to actions that are destructive, wicked, or large in scope. Small actions of selfishness, ranging from personal intolerance, impoliteness, and greed, to selfish spirituality or thinking in "me" terms, all detract from goodness in the same way.

Selfishness is often incorporated into areas of life where it does not belong, causing us to focus too intensely on ourselves, blurring the line between our wants and our needs. The selfish mind thinks in "me" terms, spawning negative emotions and traits, such as jealousy, and greed. For the selfish person, everything is "all about me." They believe statements like the following: "My way of doing things is the only right way; my religion is the only right one; my family is the most important; my problems are the worst; my life matters most." This type of thinking hinders goodness by causing pain, separation, ill will, and suffering.

~ Selfish to Selfless ~

Every person has the ability to think and act with selflessness, and each of us can find more ways to do so. Obviously, some people will choose not to act selflessly toward you; however, you cannot use that as an excuse to act selfishly.

Since you have lived through unique circumstances and experiences, your personal self-preservation is something you must figure out for yourself. Look at your life thoroughly and think about what you have, and what you have to give.

> ➢ Are you as selfless as you could be?
> ➢ Are you able to objectively view yourself and find room for improvement?
> ➢ How elaborate do your material possessions need to be?
> ➢ Do you look down on others?
> ➢ Are you intolerant or envious of others?

Think about these questions and add more of your own. Be willing to accept the fact that you may have some work to do in order to become more selfless.

Like any living thing, we must focus on our needs in order to survive. But unlike other creatures, we have the ability to differentiate between what we want and what we need. Often, we know what we need, but still want excessively beyond that point, and are all guilty of this to one extent or another. Thoughts and actions are personal choices, so no one can make them, correct them, or account for them except you. Bring more goodness into the world by changing selfish thoughts, emotions, and actions into selfless ones.

✓ To Do List: Look Within to Change

❑ **Understand why selfishness exists:**

➢ Wired in the mind for physical survival.

❑ **Understand why selflessness exists:**

➢ Wired in the mind for higher levels of self-preservation that are as important as the physical aspects of survival, if not more so.

❑ **Encourage your selfless instincts.**

➢ Identify selfish thoughts and behaviors, large and small:

➢ Do not rationalize you are not selfish simply because you have not broken any laws or committed significant actions of selfishness.

➢ Recognize that selfishness covers everything from physically hurting someone, to intolerance, to stealing, to making fun of someone.

❑ **Selfishness can be changed:**

➢ Foster goodness by replacing selfishness with selflessness.

❑ **Make a personal to-do list to encourage selflessness:**

Notes — Look Within:

Notes — Look Within:

CHAPTER 6

SELFISH TO SELFLESS

Only a life lived for others is a life worthwhile."
—Albert Einstein

Why does it seem like such a struggle for people to be selfless? Even though we inherently know being selfless is a moral, virtuous thing, many people fail to act selflessly to their full potential. The reasons for this shortcoming are many: we can choose to be selfish; we may have forgotten how to be selfless; or maybe haven't even considered it.

Do you think you are selfish? Do you *know* you are and honestly admit, "It's all about me," and believe that's okay? For many people, any type of giving, sharing, or patience beyond personal needs can be a challenge at times (myself included). The road to selflessness will be traveled every day of your life because it requires daily effort and maintenance. This road can be bumpy and difficult to navigate, and you may make some wrong turns along the way or get lost from time to time, but you can always find your way back.

Treating others with selflessness is not a new idea, but one that is often ignored. People can be so busily involved with *their* lives, *their* troubles, and *their* wants, making it difficult to accommodate even the smallest actions of selflessness. Without those small actions, hope inevitably wanes for selfless thoughts and actions on a grander scale. When hope is gone, excessive negativity is all but formally invited into our lives, funneling us into a downward spiral of negativity affecting individuals, families, organizations, and even entire countries. Changing that downward spiral is such an enormous task that we can try to rationalize and justify being selfish by believing we are helpless to affect change on our own. After all, what can one person do to stem the tide of selfishness in our world?

The truth is far more hopeful, however. When people become selfless, tiny seeds of goodness are planted and begin to grow. Sometimes goodness grows subtly, but it also grows exponentially. A little selflessness goes a long way toward bringing our world back to good, and each of us can help. To start, reflect on how you may neglect to treat others as you should. Are you as kind or courteous as you could be? Do you become quick to anger, or find your patience wears thin easily? Are slight inconveniences blown out of proportion and handled in a selfish manner?

In order to get back to good, acknowledge and become aware of your selfish tendencies. I have developed a simple self-assessment for you to determine where you fit on a selfish/ selfless scale. This assessment will enable you to see what you need to do in order to bring more selflessness into your life. The following definitions and categories will help your determine your level of selfishness. Everyone fits somewhere between the extremes of being purely selfless and purely selfish, but there is room for improvement no matter where you fit.

***

The following definitions are by no means all-inclusive. Please add your own insights to them.

***

~ Defining Selflessness ~

Selflessness, by definition, is the nature of people who are truly generous individuals, putting the needs of others first. They will give to anyone, at any time, often surrendering or sacrificing something of their own in the process. They realize nothing in life is truly their own, and offer help, kindness, and material assistance to the best of their ability.

Selfless people give because they inherently know giving is the right thing to do. They do not give to receive attention or because they expect something in return. Their selfless acts range from being courteous while driving to giving donations; from volunteering time to taking the first steps in order to repair a broken relationship. In addition, they give as freely to those they do not know as to loved ones.

Another trait of selfless people is tolerance. They will not judge based on appearance, spiritual beliefs, race, or preconceived ideas or stereotypes, and offer respect to everyone. They will not look down on another person regardless of social, economic, or educational class because they choose to apply the fact that everyone is equal.

Genuinely selfless people are forgiving and readily offer apologies by not holding grudges and putting aside personal pride if it means helping someone or mending a broken relationship. Finally, selfless people are genuinely nice, approachable, warm, and friendly. They offer patience in situations where most people would become angry. Rather than becoming impatient, they offer encouragement. Kindness is always a companion to their giving, and recipients of their selflessness never feel something is owed.

~ Defining Selfishness ~

Selfish people are those who care about themselves to the exclusion of others, but this definition goes far beyond simple self-centeredness to encompass all selfish thoughts and behaviors. Selfish people live in a clouded bubble, dealing exclusively with what pertains to them. Blindly going about their lives, thinking only of what benefits them, they choose not to see selflessness as necessary and good. Rarely will they look outside their bubble, and when they do, their perceptions are as blurry and distorted as if they were looking through a real bubble.

Selfish people cannot comprehend why a person would give to someone without being forced to do so. They believe in the necessity of gaining something for any act of giving. In other words, they only give in order to receive. This perspective causes them to tend exclusively to what affects *them,* inside of *their* bubble. Unfortunately, they never pop the bubble or find a way to give to others outside of it.

As selfish people sit in their self-inflicted confines, a distorted view of reality affects every aspect of life. Self-centeredness causes them to become too close to their lives, material belongings, and problems (which are often mere inconveniences). This begins the "it's all about me" complex. Even if life is going well, they find something to complain about. If life happens to place some bumps in the road, their complaints turn into tantrums.

As selfishly minded people gain more material possessions, success, perceived power, or status, they always want more, and are rarely satisfied or thankful for what they have. At some point, selfishness affects the lives of those around them. They may look at others who have received a blessing, be it in family, money, or success, and go so far as to begrudge the recipient of that blessing.

The selfish mind tends to think negatively, "No one should have anything if I don't. I should not be made to suffer, struggle, or do without unless everyone else shares the same fate." They cannot enjoy someone else's happiness and good fortune because they always want more for themselves. Instead of taking a thankful perspective, selfish people are trapped in a circle of negativity where they constantly worry about what others may be getting or have received. They feel shorted, cheated, and slighted by life, society, and other people.

Selfish people show an amazing amount of intolerance, ranging from ignorance and impoliteness to prejudice, spite, or hatred based on racial, social, educational, or spiritual differences. They feel superior to others to superficial, egotistical reasons and often feel they have to tolerate other people. When dealing with others, they may act aggressively or be condescending, because the selfish mind can have much brain but very little mind. Translation: a selfish person can be well versed and successful in the practical areas of life, but may lack and ignore the knowledge of how to treat others with goodness.

Of course, selfish people will not see their own faults or mistakes because for this type of mindset, it truly is "all about me." Remember, you do not have to commit terrible actions or do great harm to others to be considered a selfish individual. Caring exclusively for your needs can taint you with selfishness.

~ Selfless/Selfish Levels ~

Now that you have general definitions of selflessness and selfishness, we will begin organizing those definitions into a scale with different groups so you can assess your own placement. Levels can be separated into five general categories, open to your personal interpretation, and are as follows:

1. Completely Selfless = Goodness
2. Generally Selfless = Givers
3. Selfishly Selfless = Givers and Takers
4. Selfish = Takers
5. Excessive / Evil Selfishness = Evil Takers

At one end of the scale lies the ideal goodness of complete selflessness, and the other end is the extreme of excessive, evil selfishness. Everyone thinks and acts in ways that put them at some point on the scale. Place yourself into the level or levels that best describes you. Once you have a point of reference, you can begin to work toward becoming more selfless. Remember, you may need objective opinions from people who know you in order to make an accurate placement. Consult those who know you well; ask them to offer opinions and candid observations in order to help you assess your proper category.

#1: Completely Selfless-Goodness

Complete selflessness is more of an ideal, rather than an attainable level of human ability. However, an extremely small percentage of humanity manages to fit into this category by consistently sustaining a lifestyle that entails giving to others in thought, action, and attitude. They live for others, understanding and showing the true meaning of life: to give, to be helpful, to show tolerance and care, to offer forgiveness, and to live with goodness. Their thoughts and deeds are selflessly directed toward others, as well as the very nature that supports life. Selfish actions, beyond basic needs of survival, are non-existent.

#2: Generally Selfless — Givers

This level describes people who exemplify traits that define selflessness. They consistently offer themselves to others in any capacity possible. While the vast majority of their thoughts and actions are selfless, emotions, feelings, and circumstances in life can cause this type of person to lose their way from selflessness from time to time, although very rarely. A person in this category would never intentionally hurt, harm, or cause pain. More than likely, people who truly belong in this category would not place themselves in it, as they always feel they could be more doing more to be selfless.

#3: Selfishly Selfless — Givers & Takers

The vast majority of humanity belongs in this level, which contains aspects of selflessness and selfishness. People who fit in this level care for themselves and the needs and wants of others, but are not selfless to their full potential. They are well-meaning, good-natured, and caring people who simply do not live as selflessly as they could. At times, selfless thoughts and actions may only apply to those who are important to them, such as family and friends, while they show something less than selflessness toward others (or vice versa).

Selfishly selfless people can be judgmental and hurtful. Examples range from getting upset over the everyday situations of life to holding grudges; from maintaining a view of superior or exclusively righteous beliefs to showing slight amounts of prejudice toward those who are different. They may believe any perspective differing from theirs is incorrect, invariably resulting in some degree of intolerance and judgment. However, this person will never tolerate the extremes of hatred or violence.

On the flip side, they are selfless by giving to others, offering help, kindness, forgiveness, and showing genuine concern and compassion. Remember, the majority of humanity fits somewhere into this level, with ample room for improvement.

#4: Selfish — Takers

This category covers people who care exclusively for themselves. They often lead socially correct lives, function well in society, and become materially successful by caring for what is important to them. However, everything in life is "all about them." They only look for ways to benefit themselves, protect what is "theirs" to an unreasonable degree, and do not care for the needs, feelings, or wishes of a person who is outside their perspective.

A selfish person does not consider giving to others for the sake of goodness, and can be intolerant and judgmental. If your beliefs are not like theirs, then you are wrong. If you are not in the same social, racial, or educational class, they will look down on you, be intolerant, or try to degrade you for your differences. Selfish people maintain perspectives of superiority and choose not to acknowledge the fact that people are fundamentally equal.

#5: Extreme Selfishness — Evil Takers

Those who care exclusively for themselves and break laws of humanity, society, and goodness in order to get what they desire fall into this category. They will use force, violence, deceit, or evil, heinous, or atrocious actions in order to satisfy their wants. People who fit in this level do not care if their actions will affect others. They lack and/or ignore any sense of right and wrong, do not have remorse about any harm committed, and are not affected by conscience. True spirituality is non-existent in their lives. Any perceived spirituality or connection to goodness is grossly distorted from reality (i.e. to kill in the name of a particular belief or inflict harm on others because they are not of the same spiritual faith, race, nation, or social class).

Only a relatively small percentage of humanity fits into this category. That fact may be hard to accept because of the preponderance of negativity reported in the media, but out of the billions of people inhabiting our world, only a minuscule number actually fall into this category. Unfortunately, evil actions, and the people who commit them, get inordinate amounts of attention.

~ Where Do You Fit? ~

Determine your placement. You may fit into more than one category due to the many different situations and dynamic circumstances you come across. Remember, you may have a more selfish perspective than you realize, so your assessment may not be entirely accurate. Ask people who know you well to objectively and candidly describe your traits and tendencies. Try not to get angry or defensive about their view, but consider their comments as tools for you to make a proper assessment, ultimately helping you become more selfless. The following quote may be helpful when listening to what others have to say about you.

"Honest criticism is hard to take, particularly from a relative, a friend, an acquaintance, or a stranger."

--Franklin P. Jones

If you feel you are not selfish, please reassess your thoughts and actions, past and present, and take a closer look. Maybe you are not as tolerant as you should be. For instance, does race or physical appearance play a role in how you view a person? Are you tolerant of other spiritual or religious beliefs, or think your views are exclusively correct? There are also other avenues available to explore:

> - Do you gossip?
> - Are you jealous of the possessions, lifestyle, or accomplishments of others?
> - Are you selfless only with your loved ones, but not toward other people (or vice versa)?
> - Do you outwardly show selflessness, but think the opposite?
> - Are you easily upset in situations that require patience?
> - Are you judgmental?
> - Do apologies, forgiveness, and thankfulness flow easily from your mind as well as your mouth?

Take a close, objective look at your thoughts and actions and find areas where you need improvement.

~ Become Selfless ~

How did your personal assessment go? After identifying problem areas, make a list of your selfish thoughts and actions — don't forget the small things. Draft a plan to correct selfish tendencies by writing down what you can do in order to change and promptly put that plan into action. Remember, moving to selflessness is a process that takes effort and time. Start small and be consistent in your approach.

Simple daily actions, such as smiling and saying hello to someone walking by or being genuinely nice to others are a great start. You can hold a door for someone, be patient while driving, offer an apology, and make the first call to repair a relationship. Say thank you. Hold your temper. Give of yourself in any number of different ways to people you know, as well as to those you don't. Giving selflessly can be accomplished by sharing kindness, forgiveness, tolerance, patience, time, encouragement, compassion, and material help, to name just a few.

Many people consider themselves to be selfless, but they can be quick to balk or stop short when an opportunity to be kind or giving to others is presented to them. They may have difficulty extending even the smallest actions of selflessness, such as leaving a generous tip at a restaurant, saying thank you, offering to pay for something, giving tolerance, or showing kindness and patience in everyday actions. They can be self-centered regarding faith and forget that true spirituality demands goodness, selflessness, *and* tolerance.

Do not let this become the case for you. Be less concerned with telling others how selfless you are and let your actions be your voice. Small measures of selflessness are just as important as grand ones because they build the foundation for becoming a more giving, selfless person.

When you wander from the path of goodness (and we all will), your selfless acts can lose value. For instance, if someone gives to you in some way, yet treats you badly in other ways, their selfless acts can lose value. Therefore, it is especially important to be as consistent as possible with selfless behaviors. Of course, there will be times when you fall short and make mistakes — being selfless is not always easy. If you wander from the path, be sure to find your way back to it. Remember, "Success consists of getting up just one more time than you fall." *–Oliver Goldsmith*

~ Only Judge *Your* Selfishness ~

Many people self-righteously label those who are well off in some area of life as being selfish. Who is able to draw the distinction between what is too much and just enough as it pertains to lifestyle or possessions? For example, a person who earns an average wage and owns a modest house may believe a person with a substantial home has "too much". To that person, "too much" may mean someone who owns lavish houses on two continents, a 300-foot yacht, and other materialistic luxuries. However, to a person struggling to put food on the table and pay the rent, the person with a modest house may seem to have "too much." Finally, a person who has given up most of his worldly possessions to selflessly help others may view everyone who does not give to that same degree as having "too much." This begs the question: Who can definitively judge what is considered too much?

How much does one person need? Only that one person can answer this question. No one has the right to say what is too much or incorrect regarding the material possessions or lifestyles, as long as no hurt or harm is caused. You may express what would be correct for yourself, but you should not judge other people — that is not an action of goodness.

Material possessions and lifestyle, as long as they cause no hate, harm, or intolerance, are a matter of perspective and personal choice. (That's not to say those choices are spiritually or morally correct, I am merely pointing out that you and I do not have the right to judge.) Every person is responsible for deciding his or her actions and every individual is ultimately held accountable for those actions. Again, do not judge others — apply judgment to yourself and choose to find more goodness in your life.

Do not automatically stereotype an individual as selfish simply because of financial means. Wealth, in and of itself, is not necessarily an indicator of selfishness. Actions toward others are. A person who is well off financially can be as kind, generous, and giving as a person who has means that are more modest. Indeed, people of modest means can be as stingy, self-centered, and selfish as the night is dark. Learn to look at a person's attitude of selflessness instead of looking at what he or she owns.

***

Having a selfless attitude toward others is far more important than wealth or material possessions.

***

Concern yourself with your choices instead of judging the actions and possessions of others. Ultimately, you justify and account for *your* thoughts, actions, and lifestyle — no one else's. Act with selflessness and tolerance, instead of passing judgment.

~ Be Selfless ~

Being selfless will help you find purpose in life. Take a step back from the life you are given and realize you may be selfish at times. It may be difficult for you to recognize selfish thoughts and behaviors, but do not let this discourage you — let it motivate you to learn how to recognize and shun selfishness.

Any selfless act, whether giving something you own, offering a nice gesture, or being tolerant, will expand and grow exponentially as it touches the lives of others. A single act of selflessness, done for the sake of goodness, will give rise to more good thoughts and deeds. Everyone you come in contact with can be inspired in such beneficial ways that the overall positive effects are nearly impossible to imagine. Become selfless to the best of your ability.

✓ To Do List: Selfish to Selfless

❑ **Assess your thoughts and actions.**

❑ **Rate yourself on the selfish/selfless scale:**
  ➢ Get an objective opinion to help you identify what you need to work on.
  ➢ List your selfish behaviors, make a plan, and commit to become selfless.

❑ **Be selfless to the best of your ability.**

❑ **Do not judge others with respect to their possessions or lifestyle, as long as no hurt or harm is caused:**
  ➢ Recognize that everyone is accountable for his or her own lifestyle and actions.

MY GOALS TO
BECOME SELFLESS

Date:_____

- _____
- _____
- _____
- _____
- _____
- _____
- _____
- _____
- _____
- _____
- _____
- _____
- _____
- _____

Notes — Selfish to Selfless:

Notes — Selfish to Selfless:

CHAPTER 7

PRACTICE GIVING

"You make a living by what you get,
but you make a life by what you give."

—Winston Churchill

The act of giving transforms selfless thoughts and aspirations directly into action. To give, in the truest sense of the word, means to do so for the sake of goodness. You should not give because you expect something in return, but because you know in your heart it is the right thing to do. As the keeper of your kindness, your tolerance, your positive attitude of gratitude, and your patience, you have the responsibility to give those things. Share them often and give freely.

While we cannot be involved in everything that occurs in our family, community, or world, most of us are able to direct a larger part of our time and energy toward giving in some way. Helping others, caring for nature, and offering tolerance and forgiveness are a few things you can do. Gifts of your patience, kindness, compassion, and empathy, as well as time, money, encouragement, and a positive attitude are several more.

The extent to which you give makes little difference on the scales of goodness. The important thing is for you *to give*. For instance, if you are only able to donate a small amount of money or time, do not fret — give what you can at this moment. Give what you can when you can, because the act of giving is what's important.

~ Give Tolerance ~

"No one is born hating another person because of the color of his skin, or his background, or his religion. People must learn to hate; and if they can learn to hate they can be taught to love, for love comes more naturally to the human heart than its opposite."

-Nelson Mandela

Diversity is a law of nature, and the diversity of humanity is worthy of tolerance. People naturally feel comfortable with things that are familiar to them. That being said, we should be very tolerant of one another despite our superficial differences, as we are essentially the same. Our meager genetic differences are what give us variations in skin color, height, and other physical characteristics. Add to these our cultural, spiritual, and personal distinctions, and we still have no justification for intolerance.

No human being has the right to dictate what should be tolerated regarding beliefs, characteristics, lifestyles, or perspectives, as long as those things do not promote hatred or harm. Simply because a person is different from you in some way does not give you the right or justification to be intolerant of that diversity. By the same token, you must not feel superior or better than someone else because of differences. There are many ways to live that may differ from the ways you choose, and they each can be as valid as yours. The beauty of our world stems from the very diversity that exists within it.

Intolerance encompasses everything from disliking someone because of looks, such as race, dress, or physical appearance, to being intolerant of a person's beliefs, lifestyle, or personality, and does not have to be outwardly expressed to be hurtful. When you harbor intolerant thoughts, they affect your outlook and attitude, eventually causing selfishness and negativity to be expressed through words and actions, even if you are not consciously aware of it. When you are intolerant of others for any reason, you are also intolerant of yourself.

"Everyone comes from the same source. If you hate another human being, you're hating part of yourself."

-Elvis Presley

~ Personal Tolerance ~

Every individual has distinctive viewpoints and opinions resulting from unique beliefs, personalities, and life experiences. While your views, perspectives, and opinions are correct and true for you, they are not necessarily the best or most righteous, simply your own. Problems develop when you think your views are superior or exclusively correct and try to force them onto others.

Try not to think your point of view is irrefutably correct or your beliefs are exclusively right, because thinking this way stems from a selfish perspective. This is exemplified very well by what I like to call the "I'm the only one who knows how to drive!" syndrome.

Driving is a most useful example for demonstrating the self-centeredness of people because it so readily brings out undesirable tendencies. There is nothing like getting behind the wheel of a car to bring out impatience, selfishness, anger, self-righteousness, and intolerance; but the principles demonstrated can apply to every aspect of life.

"I'm the only one who knows how to drive!"

When you drive down the road, you tend to see *your* immediate needs and no one else's. You may believe other travelers do not need to get where they are going as badly as you do. Their right to be on the road is definitely not as important as yours. *You* have to do what *you* have to do in order for *you* to get to where *you* are going. Do you see a pattern here?

Syndrome Example 1: Imagine you are in a hurry, but the car in front of you is going the speed limit or perhaps a little faster. Does that driver's "slow driving" begin to irritate you? Do you start to tailgate the car, thinking, "C'mon! Can't you see I'm in a hurry? SPEED UP!" After a stoplight or stop sign, you may think the driver is taking an extraordinarily long time to get going — maybe just to tick you off a little bit.

Now, anger and intolerance have entered the picture. That person could drive faster! After all, *your* need to reach *your* destination is more important than another driver's right to observe the speed limit, because *your* needs come first. Think about why you are angry. What is the other person doing that's wrong? How would you feel if you were treated with this same type of intolerance?

Turn the example around: You've had a rough day. In order to relax and unwind, you plan to take a nice, leisurely ride home. You are traveling at the speed limit or perhaps a little faster when you notice a pair of headlights in the rearview mirror. The light becomes increasingly brighter as the car gets closer…and closer still. Finally, it is so close that a tap of your brake pedal would certainly cause a collision. What is this driver doing? What a jerk! Some people are so impatient! Your right to drive the speed limit is more important than the tailgater's desire to get to his destination faster. Once again, your needs are more important, and your perspective is exclusively correct.

Do you remember the first part of the example? Is it okay if you are intolerant or impatient with someone else when it suits your needs, but not okay when those things are done to you? If you recognize yourself in these situations, take the opportunity to identify and address your actions and attitudes. Try on the other person's driving gloves and view things for a minute from his perspective.

Syndrome Example 2: This scenario starts when you are driving down the open road. Suddenly, someone turns in front of you. You have to slam on the brakes to avoid a collision. To top things off, the inconsiderate driver seems to be taking forever to get up to speed. You tailgate the bumper to make sure he knows you are upset and think, "That unbelievable "#@*&!@#$*^&% so-and-so!" Your blood pressure is up, you are upset, and the way you are driving unquestionably shows your anger. "What an inconsiderate driver! He is definitely wrong," you say (possibly with a little stronger language).

While that may be true, you should remember to give that driver some space. "Why should I?" you may ask. "A driver should know better! This is my lane! That's unacceptable! A driver like that shouldn't be allowed on the road."

First of all, relax! There is no reason to become upset, territorial, or impatient over petty things as quickly as many people do. Everybody makes mistakes. Have patience. Be tolerant and understanding about the mistakes of others because you want and deserve that same tolerance for yourself — don't you? Learn to give people the benefit of the doubt and treat the shortcomings and mistakes of others with the same amount of tolerance you afford yourself.

Turn this second example around: If you were to pull out in front of someone thinking you had plenty of time to do so, but really didn't, you would undoubtedly appreciate another driver giving you some slack (tolerance). How would you feel if the driver you just cut off were to flash the bright lights and crawl up your bumper? Do *they* then become "the jerk?" Do you think, "Can't they understand? I thought I had more time. I just made an error in judgment! What an impatient "&^%#*!" In other words, do you give the same amount of patience and understanding to others you afford yourself?

***

Apply these principles to every aspect of life and recognize your actions of intolerance. Give the same amount of patience, tolerance, and understanding to others that you want for yourself.

***

Now that you have had the opportunity to think about these scenarios, consider the following questions. Do you often blame *"They - Them - Him - Her – She – He - It?"* Is someone or something else always at fault? Do you notice everyone else has faults and makes bad mistakes? You may think, "I don't make many mistakes or have many faults. Well, at least mine are not as bad as other peoples'." While your mistakes and faults may not seem so bad, that's because they do not seem so bad to you. When you only have tolerance for yourself, you immediately become intolerant of others.

Do you dislike certain ways people treat you, only to turn around and act the same way? Are you able to find justification for your mistakes easily? Do you readily offer tolerance for the shortcomings of others? Ask yourself these questions and answer them honestly. Ironically, the worst perpetrators of personal intolerance are often the most inept dealing with intolerance aimed at them.

Many of us feel other people are often at fault, wrong, or misguided. This is demonstrated when we are too critical of the shortcomings and mistakes of others, while forgetting or minimizing our own weaknesses and errors. Instead, take the high-powered binoculars of criticism that so deftly point out the faults of others and view yourself through them. You will see that you have just as many imperfections (if not more). Accept the fact that you are no better than the person next to you. When you recognize this, you will find it harder to feel intolerant of others.

~ **Spiritual Tolerance** ~

Spirituality is a very personal and deep-rooted issue, and discussing differing views often leads to intense debates, disagreements, or arguments. Spiritual convictions are often so strong and profound, that we can find it virtually impossible to tolerate and respect different outlooks. Nevertheless, living with goodness dictates that we become as tolerant as possible in every aspect of our existence, especially those concerning spiritual beliefs.

People naturally view things differently, but spiritual views can easily become selfishly skewed. Problems begin to surface when people try to force their convictions on others. Remember, just as there are many different languages, many different ways to set up governments, and many ways to exhibit culture, there can be many interpretations of religious and spiritual beliefs.

If you express faith in your own way, it is important to allow others to express faith in their own way, as well. To become more tolerant, spend time exploring other views of faith. The task of fostering goodness is more important than arguing about which belief is the only "right" one. Focus your energy on what truly matters — connecting spiritually in order to foster goodness.

"There was a time I used to reject those who were not of my faith. Now my heart has grown capable of taking on many forms: a pasture for gazelles, a convent for Christians, a temple for idols, a Kaaba for the pilgrim, a table for the Torah, a book of the Koran.

*My religion is love - whichever the route love's caravan shall take,
that path shall be the path of my faith."*

**-Muhyiddin Ibn 'Arabi
(1165-1240)**

Countless belief systems, traditions, and perspectives can be valid as long as they do not promote hateful, intolerant, or harmful behaviors. You may not know about differing beliefs or feel completely comfortable with other spiritual customs or views, but spiritual tolerance does not ask you to believe or worship differently. Spiritual tolerance simply asks you to be open to the fact that people connect in their own way. You are doing no disservice to your faith by being tolerant of other beliefs. On the contrary, being tolerant is an act of goodness that true faith expects and requires from you.

~ Become Tolerant ~

Find ways to stem the tide of intolerance in your mind. If you are intolerant of the outward appearance of another person, remind yourself that others must tolerate the way you look. If you do not like the personality or beliefs of another person, remember, your personality and beliefs have to be tolerated by others as well. You simply do not have the right to be intolerant because of differences.

Can someone force you to stop being intolerant? The answer is a resounding *no*. That change must come from within you. You have a choice to be tolerant of differences — it is the right thing to do. Remember, if you take a tolerant view, there is no guarantee others will do the same for you. In the real world, you will face intolerance in some form. Be a better person and show tolerance to the best of your ability.

~ Give Help ~

"In helping others, we shall help ourselves, for whatever good we give out completes the circle and comes back to us."

-Flora Edwards

There is a constant ebb and flow throughout the world regarding what people have, what people need, and what people have to give. We can be strong at times, yet weak or helpless under different circumstances. Out of that imbalance comes our responsibility and opportunity to help one another.

The ways we can help are one another are as vast and varied as the number of people on Earth, because each of us can help in unique ways. These range from giving time or money to being genuinely kind; from helping a troubled youth to showing compassion; from lending a sympathetic ear to adopting a child, as well as everything in between. Some people feel comfortable volunteering to benefit a specific cause, while others give by donating time or expertise through large organizations. Still others can help by writing a check, which is volunteering in a different way. No form of help is too big or too small.

When some aspects of life are going well, as when you may be enjoying good health, stable finances, or good cheer, share some of that good fortune by directing it toward other people. If life is not going so well, try to give even if you feel you cannot. When you don't have time to give, find another way, such as giving money or kindness. All means of giving are important.

While each person shares the responsibility to be helpful, we are not destined to give in the same way. Do not measure your gifts of help against the gifts of others; give to the best of *your* ability. Help may go to family members and people you come across daily, as well as to others you may not know in more distant places. Learn to offer help because you want to, because it fosters goodness, not because you expect to gain from it. Do not brag about any help you have given, or make a recipient of your helpfulness feel they owe you. When you help someone, you are fulfilling a part of your responsibility for goodness.

~ Give Forgiveness ~

"If we really want to love,
we must learn how to forgive."

-Mother Teresa

To forgive is to let go, to choose to replace feelings of anger and hurt with the calmness and peace of mind forgiveness affords. Forgiveness can change negative feelings, emotions, and actions into positive thoughts and attitudes. Undoubtedly, there are times when forgiving is hard, but the benefits far outweigh any difficulties involved. Forgiveness can repair relationships, remove stress and negativity, and move you closer to goodness.

Over the course of life, every one of us will become hurt or angered by the words, thoughts, and actions of other people or by forces of nature. When you are hurt or angry, you move through a natural process to deal with those feelings. Becoming mad or detached from whomever or whatever has caused your pain is normal, but those feelings may turn into grudges and breed negativity in your attitude, well-being, and treatment of others.

The act of forgiveness is a way to release negativity, but it may be difficult. Pain can run so deep or be so scarring emotionally, that releasing a grudge and offering forgiveness may not be the first thing that comes to mind when you are hurt and angered. Remember, there are no timetables or specific steps you can take to hasten forgiveness, because subtle and major differences affect every situation and person in unique ways.

~ Types of Forgiveness ~

Type I Forgiveness — Forgive *and* Forget: The defining characteristics of Type I Forgiveness allow you to harness the positive power of forgiveness to continue in a healthy, productive relationship with someone who may have hurt, offended, or harmed you. Many different factors can either help or hinder Type I Forgiveness, the most important of which is your attitude and ability to forgive. If you are a forgiving person by nature and can shrug off negativity quite easily, forgiving and forgetting will come naturally for you. However, if you have trouble letting go and offering forgiveness readily, you may have a tougher time. Extremely difficult circumstances and situations often cannot simply be forgiven and forgotten. In these cases you will need to explore a different type of forgiveness.

Type II Forgiveness — Forgive *to* Forget: Sometimes situations are so difficult that you cannot simply forgive and forget. Your hurt, pain, and anger can be so devastating that forgiving and forgetting is virtually impossible. Maybe the person who caused your pain is unwilling or unable to offer an apology or doesn't acknowledge any wrongdoing. Maybe you have lost contact, or the person has passed away. Type II Forgiveness can help you deal with situations involving other people, and it can also help you deal with circumstances and situations out of your control.

When forces of nature cause devastation, or when you or a loved one suffers physical illness, there is no one for you to specifically blame, no one who can offer you an apology. By learning to forgive and let go, you will be able to focus on your positive attitude and responsibility for goodness. When forgiving *and* forgetting is not possible, forgiving *to* forget can help you work through the negativity that is sometimes inescapable. Although you may not be able to forgive directly for any number of reasons, you are in effect forgiving by letting go of the negativity associated with certain situations. Type II Forgiveness allows you to move on in a healthier, more positive way.

~ Try to Forgive ~

With your connection to goodness, your perspective of thankfulness, and your selfless attitude, reflect on reasons why you should forgive, and try your best to do so. Remember to pay particular attention to your thankful checklist and be grateful for what you have received. Even if you cannot forgive readily or completely, it is important to keep trying. Challenge yourself to be a better person by forgiving as much and as often as you can. Of course, you will not be able to forgive readily in every circumstance, but try your best.

"Forgiveness helps you move forward. No one benefits more from forgiveness than the one who forgives."

-*Unknown*

Forgiving and releasing grudges forces negative emotions out of your mind so positive thoughts and feelings can help you foster goodness. There will be moments when other people do not understand what hurts you — sometimes they simply do not care. At other times, you will not get apologies or sincere explanations for many things that cause you pain. While people certainly cause problems, oftentimes difficult situations are just negative facts of life you must learn to deal with.

When you have trouble forgiving, remember that you have done, or will do things that offend, anger, or hurt others. If you desire forgiveness for your mistakes, forgive and release grudges to the best of your ability. When you are able to forgive, be sure to offer it in a true and complete manner. Do not hastily claim you have forgiven someone and then hold it over that person's head or make those you have forgiven feel they owe you.

～ Give Apologies ～

"An apology is the superglue of
life. It can repair just about anything."

–Lynn Johnston

Apologies can build bridges across gaps or faults in relationships and heal wounds that have been created. A true apology, by its very nature, shows you are sorry for what you have done, and just as importantly, that you do not intend to do the same thing again. When giving a sincere apology, you understand that you have brought some kind of pain or offense to someone and sincerely empathize with the hurt they feel. A true apology means you will try in earnest to stop the behavior or actions that necessitated the apology in the first place.

When you are the one who offends or causes pain, you must be the one to offer a heartfelt, sincere apology. If you have wronged someone, apologize. If a person believes you have wronged him or her, try to get to the source of the problem and offer an apology for any misunderstanding. This may not always be practical or plausible, but it can work wonders to repair relationships and bring a positive energy and attitude to all involved. And remember, simply because something would not offend or hurt you does not mean it cannot offend someone else. Be aware of what you say and do to others. If they are hurt by your words or actions, set aside your pride, apologize, and ask for forgiveness.

When you act in ways that are hurtful to others, the only way to correct the situation is to go to the person and admit what you have done was wrong. Then, offer a sincere apology, which is not simply lip service—it shows you understand and empathize with the hurt you have caused. Once you apologize, you are required to make every effort to stop the offending behavior. This step is a very important factor in repairing relationships and encouraging forgiveness. Complete forgiveness will become a more difficult process if the "wrongdoer" does not make a sincere apology.

~ Give Kindness ~

*"Kindness is the language which
the deaf can hear and the blind can see."*

-Mark Twain

Giving is complete when it is carried out with kindness, such as helping others in a caring, compassionate way, or by giving sympathy, forgiveness, and love. In other instances, kindness may be less obvious, but no less important; such as holding your anger in check — even if you have perceived the right to be angry, tempering your words to prevent an argument or backing down once one has started. Other ways to offer kindness include being polite to a person you do not really care for, expressing tolerance, and maintaining your composure and patience when dealing with the mistakes and shortcomings of others.

Acts of kindness can occur when we simply change the way we face annoying, everyday situations. We often get irritated with people who can't control the very situations that cause us grief. Usually, they are just innocent bystanders. For instance, if you are at a crowded restaurant and your food takes a long time to arrive at the table, do you become angry and take it out on the server? Do you get upset at the telephone repair technician who shows up to fix your phone line because you are angry the line is in trouble? Do you become annoyed and intolerant of others in a crowded store even though you are a contributing factor to that crowd? Ask yourself if you should be getting angry with the people involved in these circumstances. Learn to direct your irritation or anger at situations, rather than at people who just happen to be around when you become annoyed.

Giving kindness will benefit you as much as the person who receives it. Kindness brings peace and allows people to act with reason and intellect instead of reacting with selfishness and negativity. Think of examples in life where you lose patience and get angry too quickly with people who do not deserve it. By truly listening, being tolerant, saying thanks, and being patient, you can show kindness. Every kind action is grand because of the exponential potential for goodness that exists within it.

~ Give Environmentally ~

*We do not inherit the Earth from our
ancestors, we borrow it from our children.*

-Native American Proverb

Humankind has lived symbiotically with nature for millennia. Until relatively recently, that relationship has been successful. However, due to our many technical and industrial advances, the Earth is in throes of ever-increasing pain. Nature's equilibrium is out of balance because of humanity. Signs are evident now, today, but many dire problems will not be evident for many years to come.

We consume our natural resources at an alarming rate and continue to pollute and poison the very nature that sustains us. We necessarily live "in the now" to care for our needs, but must be more proactive about living for the future — so our grandchildren's grandchildren will be sustained by a healthy planet.

~ What Can be Done? ~

You can do many things to help our planet. First, educate yourself on environmental issues and support those in the political and business arenas who combat the poisoning of our world. Take it upon yourself to learn about the hundreds of different things you can do to support and nurture the environment.

Every day you can take part by recycling, preventing pollution, handling waste products properly, conserving energy and water, seeking renewable energy sources, incorporating environmentally friendly attitudes in your purchases, and reducing and reusing. Some simple things you can do are:

> ➤ Change your light bulbs to low energy cfl bulbs.
> ➤ Become a "Recycling Ambassador " at home *and* at work or school.
>   (one guy at work calls me the cardboard cop!)
> ➤ Start composting.
> ➤ Add a low-flow faucet aerator.
> ➤ Carpool, ride a bike, or walk whenever possible.
> ➤ Use rechargeable batteries.
> ➤ Stop junk mail.
> ➤ Buy paper goods made from recycled materials.

Visit www.makeyourdifference.org for great resources on this topic — simply click on the 'Give Environmentally' link. We can only ignore the poisoning of our food and water and continue to consume natural resources at the current alarming rates for so long before our actions affect everyone. Hurting and ignoring the very environment that sustains us brings distress and suffering to all.

~ Give ~

When you are willing to share with others, you have come to realize life, and all that goes with it, is a blessing. Remember, the point is not how much you are able to give, the point is *to give*. Give of yourself because you truly want to help others and foster goodness. Give to others by nurturing our environment, offering help, and being tolerant and trusting. Offer patience and forgiveness. Listen to others and encourage with kindness. If you give without kindness your giving is significantly reduced in value.

"People will not always remember what you said; people will not always remember what you did; but people will always remember how you made them feel."

-Anonymous

Once you have gained the ability to give of yourself without expectation of getting something in return, you have mastered an important purpose for life — selflessness. Do not miss an opportunity to make someone's day, week, year, or life a bit more enjoyable by showing you care. Through selfless giving, you can change someone's life!

Take care of yourself and your loved ones, take time out for yourself when you need to, and when you are able to, give, give, and then give some more. Give in any way, to any capacity. Life can be hard enough — don't make it more difficult by hindering goodness through negative thoughts and behaviors. Fulfill a major purpose of life by finding ways to give.

I am only one, but still I am one;
I cannot do everything, but still I can do something;
And just because I cannot do everything,
I will not refuse to do the something that I can do.

—**Helen Keller**

✓ To Do List: Giving

❑ **Give personal tolerance:**
  ➢ Tolerate unique viewpoints, as long as they do not cause hate or harm.
  ➢ Be as tolerant of the shortcomings of others as you are of your own.
  ➢ Do not force your views or opinions on others.

❑ **Give spiritual tolerance:**
  ➢ Accept the fact that there are many different ways of connecting to goodness.
  ➢ Do not force your spiritual views upon others.
  ➢ Practice tolerance by remembering your spiritual preference is not correct for everyone.

❑ **Find ways to identify and stop your intolerance.**

❑ **Give help to others:**
  ➢ Offering help is one of the best things you can do in life.
  ➢ Offer help in many different and unique ways.
  ➢ Do not miss an opportunity to help someone — you will need help someday.

❑ **Give forgiveness to others:**
  ➢ Replace feelings of hurt and anger by forgiving.

- ➢ Forgive as a means to release grudges that take away from your ability to foster goodness.
- ➢ Give Type II forgiveness to help you offer Type I Forgiveness.

❑ **Give Kindness to others:**
- ➢ Allow the natural trait of kindness to surface and act with kindness in your daily ife.
- ➢ Every kind action becomes grand because of the exponential potential for goodness it contains.
- ➢ Give with kindness.

❑ **Give Environmentally:**
- ➢ Do not waste precious natural resources.
- ➢ Find ways to help our environment.

❑ **Create your own To-Do list — Giving.**

❑ **Remember, *giving* is good**
- ➢ Giving fulfills you in fundamental ways that simply are not reachable by any other means.

❑ **Visit www.makeyourdifference.org to find more ways and means to give.**

- • Recommended Reading:
  - ▪ *Giving: How Each of Us Can Change the World* **by Bill Clinton**

MY GOALS
FOR GIVING

Date:_____

- _____
- _____
- _____
- _____
- _____
- _____
- _____
- _____
- _____
- _____
- _____
- _____
- _____
- _____

Notes — Practice Giving:

Notes — Practice Giving:

CHAPTER 8

NURTURE YOURSELF

"The greatest wealth is health."

-Virgil

The quote from Virgil articulates a very powerful message. Without health, life can certainly be difficult. As I mentioned earlier, health is ultimately out of our hands, but that's not to say we should wash our hands of the entire concept, as we are responsible to care for the aspects of health that are in our control. Healthy attitudes, outlooks, and behaviors make you feel good, allowing goodness to be encouraged and shared. On the other hand, not taking care of yourself causes ill health, which can nag at your body, mind, and spirit to create negative feelings, perspectives, and physical conditions.

Take stock of your health by assessing and identifying where you need to change for the better. Once you find areas needing some attention, it is time to take action. Remember, you do not have to do this alone, as help is available from many different sources. You can seek support and guidance from friends, family, books and clubs, or health care professionals.

Health is often taken for granted; while we have it, we may not give it a second thought. However, we quickly realize just how important a place good health occupies in our lives if we lose it. Take care.

~ **Nurture Your Physical Health** ~

In order to give physical assistance to others, you must feel healthy enough to do so. If you are lying ill in a hospital bed, you will not be able to offer much physical help to someone even though you can help in other ways. To that end, I cannot stress the significance of caring for your physical body enough.

Losing just a small portion of physical health will force you to notice its importance. A sprained back muscle can impair you for weeks at a time. The common cold, a headache, a toothache, or slight depression can make you suffer and long for good health. Small inconveniences like these can make you realize just how much you value and depend on feeling healthy, while a significant loss of health can really put life into perspective.

When health is lost due to something beyond your control, such as an accident or illness, life can become difficult and painful. However, it is doubly disheartening and frustrating to lose health because of your actions. While you may not be able to stop accidents from happening or change physical conditions that afflict you, be responsible for what *is* in your control — the way you treat your body. Learn to maintain good habits in order to have the best physical health possible.

Good habits are an extremely important component of health, encompassing a wide variety of factors. Eating properly, exercising, and caring for your physical condition all play a vital role. When you exercise, your brain releases endorphins that make you feel good naturally. Why? Because we are designed to be physically active — the body is healthier because of it.

Natural, healthy foods are perfectly designed to fill you with just the right amounts of energy and nutrients, allowing your body to work to its full potential. Be conscious of food choices, levels of exercise, and medical condition by incorporating healthy habits into your daily life.

While you work to improve health by living a wholesome, well-rounded lifestyle, strive also to remove habits that have detrimental effects. Physical well-being is negatively affected by a lack of exercise, excessive drinking, excessive eating, smoking, lack of sleep, too much stress, and by using drugs of all kinds. You may choose to participate in such activities, but negative habits ultimately work against you.

If you overeat, drink excessively, and do not exercise, your body will let you know it is being neglected. You may feel sick, sluggish, or nauseated, and your mental ability to focus and feel happy is diminished. Poor physical health causes low self-esteem, irritability, and other negative feelings. These negative effects work to hinder the body's natural processes and ability to heal. Long-term abuses of your body can be very costly and will eventually catch up with you.

When you need to adjust your physical condition, find a way to put that change into motion. You may be able to correct your problems alone, or perhaps will need outside assistance. Either way can work, but in both cases the key to success is you. *You* must desire change.

Consider a wide range of issues when assessing and correcting bad physical habits, such as losing weight and exercising more often to quitting smoking or drinking; from reducing stress to becoming proactive with medical care. An entire assortment of books, seminars, medical facilities, and various programs can help you achieve and maintain physical health. Loved ones and friends can also offer help and support in your efforts. All of the information and infrastructure is in place, just waiting for you to put it into action.

～ Nurture Your Spiritual Health ～

When you are spiritually healthy, you can enjoy peace of mind due to a thankful perspective and ability to find purpose for life. Spiritual well-being allows you to view life with tranquility and comfort, permitting your innate knowledge of goodness to become prevalent in thought and action.

Since spirituality is a choice, you are *choosing* to accept the responsibility for living with goodness. Basic tenets of goodness are associated with spiritual health that are not negotiable; you must not harm, hurt, hate, or be intolerant of others based on race, culture, physical appearance, or differing beliefs. Incorporate selflessness into your life through your spiritual connection, and realize that caring exclusively for yourself and your needs will never bring true spiritual health.

There will be occasions when you act contrary to the goodness your spirituality requires of you. When this happens, accept the fact that you are not perfect — you are a human being bound to make mistakes. No matter how you may have stumbled in your efforts, you can always find a way back to thinking and acting with goodness. Direction can come from people, books, or any number of religious and spiritual organizations, and help is available everywhere you turn, but you have to make the choice to seek it out.

~ Nurture Your Emotional Health ~

Emotions play a vital role — they allow you to process experiences and help you cope and come to terms with events in your life, both good and bad. Failing to control or direct your emotions can create undesirable thoughts and behaviors that may eventually lead to poor emotional health. Achieving and maintaining emotional health is necessary in your life before you can persuasively encourage and uplift others. If you are depressed, it will be difficult enough for you to maintain a positive, thankful outlook, let alone to pass those views onto others.

Emotions can easily overcome rational, logical thoughts and actions. For instance, if you are angry or sad, those emotions can cause you to do or say things you normally would not. Negative emotions misdirect your focus and take away from your ability to foster goodness. When emotions are uncontrolled, you may to act in ways you come to regret. Learn how to deal with emotions effectively and try not to let them overwhelm your rationale and positive perspective.

I've had personal battles with depression and know firsthand of the devastating effects it can have on your life as well as affect those closest to you. Even though life can be challenging, you are ultimately in control of your emotional health; however, if you need help, find a way to address that challenge—you do not have to find it or fix it alone. Help is available. Seek it out and use it for your benefit. One important point to remember is that a fine line separates emotional health from mental health. If you know of someone who may need help, go to him or her with encouragement and understanding and find a way to offer assistance.

Emotional well-being brings positive feelings of thankfulness, happiness, care, and love. These feelings allow you to focus on life in beneficial ways, helping you promote goodness. Do your best to maintain a positive attitude in everything you do.

~ Nurture Your Financial Health ~

When finances are out of order, nearly every aspect of health can be negatively affected, causing physical symptoms of stress ranging from anxiety to nervousness to trouble sleeping. You may feel enormous pressure on your shoulders from financial worry.

***

Often, financial troubles are of our own making, so we make a complicated situation worse by adding a sense of guilt and despair.

***

There is always a way out of the stranglehold of financial trouble. In order to find your way back to good financial health, honestly address your situation. The first step is to make wise choices when spending and purchasing. If you have problems with debt, seek advice and information. Do not be ashamed if your financial house is not in order. There is always light at the end of the tunnel — but first you must enter the tunnel. The only way to do that is to take control of your financial position.

You can seek guidance from family, friends, any number of books on the topic, or by legal means. Remember, a bad financial position is not the end of the world, but an opportunity to fix up, renovate, and start anew. Once you begin, you will dramatically lighten the burden you carry and ease the amount of stress you feel. Then, you will be able to treat others with more care, respect, and understanding.

~ Health of Conscience ~

"There is no witness so terrible, no accuser so powerful as conscience which dwells within us."

-Sophocles

A conscience that is not clear leads to a mind that is not clear. When your conscience bothers you, it negatively affects health. The energy that could be used to do something positive for yourself and others is wasted with feelings of guilt, sadness, anger, or anxiousness. If you fail to clear your conscience, you are forced to carry a heavy burden, ultimately affecting your mind, spirit, and overall health.

Do you suffer from conscience pests? Conscience pests are those thoughts that creep from your conscience into your mind, where they nag you. They detract from your well-being by ruining concentration and focus and can literally eat at you from the inside out. For instance, have you ever hurt or angered someone? You know you should apologize, but until you do, your conscience nags at you. Do you worry when you promise to do something, but consistently put it off? Does a person deserve your forgiveness, yet you are not able to offer it? Should you say thanks to someone who has helped you in some way? Do you want to call a long-lost friend with whom you have lost touch, yet have not done so? Have you been selfish and resistant to change — even though your conscience is telling you differently? Have you committed hurtful, selfish, or destructive actions? Try to think of more conscience pests to add to this list.

If you have to spend time and energy repeatedly wrestling conscience pests, work to clear them out of your mind by taking action to resolve the issues once and for all. Once the negativity is out of the way, the path is clear for you to redirect that energy into more positive thoughts, attitudes, and actions. You may muffle conscience pests for years, but you will not be able to ignore them forever.

Distractions from your conscience make you lose focus on your responsibility to think and act with goodness. Let go of pride, anger, and guilt, and work to clear those pests out of your mind. Identify what you need to fix and take it upon yourself to make it right. Do not wait until it is too late. Clear your conscience now. In an instant you can lose your opportunity to make amends forever. The everyday pressures of life give you more than enough to worry about, and you should not have to deal with self-inflicted, preventable stress or ill feelings. Let your conscience be your guide and heed the messages it gives you. It is designed to let you know what is right.

"When your intelligence don't tell you something ain't right, your conscience gives you a tap on the shoulder and says hold on."

-Elvis Presley

~ Take Care ~

Good health gives you the ability to foster the most goodness possible. While this chapter does not give specific directions to maintain health, it does illustrate the importance of overall health in your efforts to promote goodness. The ways you choose to care for your health are personal decisions, but the desire and motivation ultimately comes from you. Many effective means are available to assist and guide you if you actively seek good health and commit to maintain it. Remember to be thankful for the health you have, and put it to good use by fostering goodness throughout your life. Take care.

✓ To Do List: Nurture Yourself

❑ **Improve and maintain physical health:**
  ➢ Make healthy choices and incorporate exercise into your daily routine.
  ➢ Care for medical conditions.
  ➢ Limit bad influences on the body.
  ➢ Seek help to maintain your physical health when necessary.

❑ **Improve and maintain spiritual health:**
  ➢ Strengthen spiritual health.
  ➢ Do not harm, hurt, or be intolerant of others.

❑ **Improve and maintain emotional health:**
  ➢ Control your emotions so they don't overrule your thoughts and actions.
  ➢ Stay positive in your focus on life.
  ➢ Help others maintain emotional health.

❑ **Improve your financial condition.**
  ➢ Make wise financial choices.
  ➢ If you need assistance, get advice, information, and a helping hand from family, friends, or professionals.

❑ **Clear your conscience:**
  ➢ Find and fix things that weigh upon the health of your conscience.

➢ Take action to resolve any issues you are responsible for — before it's too late.

❑ **Improve and maintain all aspects of health to the best of your ability.**

❑ **Use your health to foster goodness.**

❑ **List and work to clear your conscience pests.**

- **Recommended Reading:**
  - ➢ *Body for Life* **by Bill Phillips**
  - ➢ *Eating for Life* **by Bill Phillips**

MY GOALS FOR
BETTER HEALTH

Date:_____

- _____
- _____
- _____
- _____
- _____
- _____
- _____
- _____
- _____
- _____
- _____
- _____
- _____

Notes — Nurture Yourself:

Notes — Nurture Yourself:

Chapter 9

Finding Purpose

"Life's most urgent question is:
What are you doing for others?"

—Dr. Martin Luther King, Jr.

Whether we know it or not, we instinctively search for meaning. The way to fulfill this need is universally similar for every person, and at the same time, every individual must do so in his or her own way. Different aspects of life must be satisfied to find and fulfill purpose. For instance, having faith is not enough if you only care for your needs. Being thankful without being selfless is not enough. Being selfless without a connection to goodness is not enough. Caring for your needs exclusively is not enough. Achieving balance between your needs and selfless responsibilities can help you find complete purpose.

When you are able to manage your needs and concerns, engage in successful relationships, reach your goals, and enjoy life, you may be fulfilling certain areas of purpose. However, those areas alone are not enough to find complete meaning. You must make an effort to live with goodness, maintain a thankful perspective, give selflessly to others, and attain your goals.

In order to survive and care for yourself, your loved ones, and your future, it is necessary to engage in a lifestyle you can directly benefit from. That is a fact. Your goals may include achieving a satisfying lifestyle and caring for you and yours. The desire to feel secure earning your living, anticipating a bright future, and caring for your needs is normal, natural, and necessary, but these things alone will not allow you to find complete meaning.

You have a greater purpose for life than simply succeeding with your endeavors and goals. While you may feel good when achieving goals and dreams, if they are only associated with material possessions, accomplishments, and titles, you will ultimately learn that those things mean very little in the end. When you only accomplish materialistic and self-serving goals, you may be satisfied for a period of time but something will be missing, and no matter how much you cram into your life, a void will remain. One way to fill this emptiness is by living with goodness and selflessness.

~ Why Be Good? ~

Fostering goodness is truly important, and doing so completes a major portion of the puzzle of life's purpose. Learn to let selfless instincts guide your actions. When you reach the end of life, the legacy that remains is in how selflessly you lived, and what you have done for others. Your thoughts and actions of goodness are what ultimately matter. A profound quote speaks to this issue: "You will find, as you look back upon your life, that the moments that stand out are the moments when you have done things for others." *-Henry Drummond*

Why am I here? What's this life for? Have you asked these questions? Maybe you think, "I want to succeed. I want a house and family. I want to make it to the top. I just want to live *my* life." However, do you ever think about what will flash before your eyes as you exhale your last breath of air?

When you draw your last breath, what will your thoughts be?

- **You probably won't be thinking about:**
  - ➢ Material possessions;
  - ➢ Accomplishments, titles, or positions you have achieved;
  - ➢ How much money is in the bank;
  - ➢ Whether or not you had the nicest home;
  - ➢ Your status or position in life.

- **You might be thinking strongly about:**
  - ➢ Your connection to Goodness (or lack thereof);
  - ➢ How you have (or have not) helped others during your life;
  - ➢ How you have (or have not) been selfless and good to others;
  - ➢ Whether or not you were tolerant and giving.

Selfless thoughts and actions, no matter how big or small, are what you will take with you. It is easy to be skeptical about my claim since there is no scientific proof to support it. I can offer no measurable data on the subject, nor can I prove it with numeric values or equations. However, it almost always becomes clear in the final moments. People who are granted a second chance after a brush with death often make giving and promoting goodness top priorities. Most people do not get a second chance. Recognize the need to live with goodness before it's too late.

~ Realize ~

Do not deprive yourself of the things you need to build a safe, secure, and enjoyable environment for you and your loved ones, but do remember to think about your responsibility for goodness. Being able to look back on life knowing you have given to others is a great feeling — a feeling greater than you can completely understand now.

Recognize your blessings and allow selfless instincts to accomplish what they are designed to do. Care for nature. Offer some of your health, time, and money by giving them to others in some way. Learn to truly share. Strive to be generous, kind, trusting, and selfless as much as you possibly can. Have faith and connect to goodness while being tolerant of the ways others do so. Be thankful for all that is in your life, become selfless, take care, and learn to give. Finally, treat others with the "Golden Rule." Find *your* purpose.

✓ To Do List: Finding Purpose

❏ **Define complete purpose for life:**
  ➢ Reflect on what complete purpose means.
  ➢ Identify and fulfill your needs.
  ➢ Incorporate goodness into your life to find meaning.

❏ **Understand that there is more than a material aspect to life:**
  ➢ Remember, you won't be worrying about material possessions or accomplishments on your deathbed.

❏ **Live with goodness by being selfless:**
  ➢ Selfless thoughts and actions, no matter how big or small, are what you will take with you.

❏ **Help fulfill your complete purpose by getting back to good:**
  ➢ Have faith.
  ➢ Connect to goodness.
  ➢ Be tolerant of the ways in which other people connect.
  ➢ Be thankful.
  ➢ Be selfless.
  ➢ Learn to give.
  ➢ Take care.
  ➢ Treat others as you want to be treated.
  ➢ Be Good.

MY PURPOSE IS

Date:_____

- _____
- _____
- _____
- _____
- _____
- _____
- _____
- _____
- People that count on me.
- _____
- _____
- _____
- _____
- _____

Notes — Finding Purpose:

Notes — Finding Purpose:

CHAPTER 10

ON YOUR WAY...

"You must be the change
you wish to see in the world."

—Gandhi

All of us are capable of bringing more goodness into the world by caring for others, our environment, and living with tolerance and kindness. We each have something good to give, whether materially or by giving a great, positive attitude. No matter what your goodness is, find a way to give some of it to others.

Do it now, while you can. Do not wait. When you give to someone out of the desire to give rather than from the need to receive, you have learned to give genuinely. Make a choice to extend goodness to others by being selfless and giving as much as possible. You may not need as much as you think you need and may not want as much as you think you want. Life is a maze that must be navigated, and the only way to reach the true end is to make choices of goodness. Be mindful of your actions, because your actions toward others return twice to you.

Simplicity is pure; simplicity is often truth. As complex and awe-inspiring as nature is, we ultimately exist for simple reasons: to have faith, tend to our lives, care for nature, and to be good to one another. Fostering goodness is a major purpose and responsibility for life. Unfortunately, this truth can be easily ignored because no one can force a person to act upon it. You can exist (sometimes quite well in a material sense) by taking care of you and yours exclusively, because living selfishly is an option you have.

The desire to get back to good is a choice you must make. If you feel living with goodness does not matter, your mind may change when drawing your last breath. Strive to be good by being kind, generous, caring, and helpful to others to the best of your ability. The fact that you are trying to live with goodness will earn rewards for you and the lives you touch.

Realize that you are equal to everyone. When you truly understand and sincerely acknowledge we are all equal, you will treat others the way they deserve to be treated — with selflessness, dignity, tolerance, respect, compassion, and kindness. You may be more successful, have more money, or be smarter than others, but in the overall picture of life those things make no difference, as everyone has the ability to offer help and teach others in unique ways.

Once again, live your life, take care of yourself and your loved ones, take time for yourself when you need to, and when you are able to — give, give, and then give some more. Give in any way, to any capacity. Give time, help, and money; give tolerance and patience; and top it off by giving kindness. Give by not gossiping or criticizing, and by truly listening to what others have to say. Share your blessings.

~ Do Your Part to Bring Goodness into our World ~

The way you start your journey back to good does not make a difference. The most important thing is *to start*. You do not have to achieve prominence or be written about in history books to reach fantastic goals of goodness. Everyday acts of being kind, helpful, or patient with others are extremely important.

Goodness affects everything in an exponential way. If you do one good thing, even something as simple as driving courteously, saying thank you, or offering material help to someone in need, you are doing good. In turn, this leads to more acts of goodness, such as repairing relationships or giving kindness, love, patience, forgiveness, and tolerance. Every good action is important, and the world will be that much better for it.

"No good act performed in the world ever dies. Science tells us that no atom of matter can ever be destroyed, that no force once started ever ends: it merely passes through a multiplicity of ever-changing phases. Every good deed done to others is a great force that starts an unending pulsation through time and eternity. We may not know it, we may never hear a word of gratitude or recognition, but it will all come back to us in some form as naturally, as perfectly, as inevitably, as echo answers to sound"

-William George Jordan

Set an example by living with goodness, but always allow others the freedom to find their own path. Remember, it means different things to different people. There are religious, cultural, social, and personal differences that are good in their own way, and each can serve in some capacity to help bring humanity back to good.

Negativity will continue even when you foster goodness. Do not let that fact hinder your efforts. Of course, there will be occasions when you are treated badly, as you may experience selfishness, intolerance, or cruelty. This is an unfortunate certainty. However, do not use it as an excuse to extend bad behaviors or thoughts toward others. Live with goodness because it is the right thing to do — not because you expect it in return.

Do not let the actions of others deter or detour *your* actions of goodness by finding effective ways to deal with negativity. Realize when you are able to deal with negative circumstances, situations, and people, and learn to know when you must remove yourself from that situation before it causes *you* to think and act negatively.

You can make the world a better place by remaining true to goodness. Of course, there will be times when you fall short and get discouraged by what others do, say, or think, so don't be too tough on yourself if you lose your way. Instead, work to find your way back to good. As I said before, you may not be able to end world hunger or bring world peace, but through your thoughts and actions of goodness, you will do your part to bring our world back to good.

What difference have you made in the world by living with goodness? The answer may be short or it may branch out and touch many lives. Only *you* can choose your answer! No one can force you to exhibit true, selfless goodness; but ultimately, you are responsible and accountable for your actions. You must be the change. Take a step back from your opinions, circumstances, and daily routines, and learn to be more tolerant, kind, and grateful. Above all, learn to live with true goodness. If your life has not fostered goodness in one form or another, then you have lived for nothing. Do you want to take that thought to the grave?

Do all the good you can,
By all the means you can,
In all the ways you can,
In all the places you can,
To all the people you can,
As long as ever you can.

—*John Wesley*

CHAPTER 11

ON OUR WAY...

*"My country is the world,
and my religion is to do good."*
—Thomas Paine

Now is the time for humanity as a whole, regardless of cultural, spiritual, and individual differences, to pull together and put goodness at the forefront of our thoughts and actions. Goodness creates strong people with integrity, honesty, righteousness, and love. This, in turn, creates loving families and the desire to care for others. As principles and actions of goodness become learned, re-learned, strengthened, and passed on, a more caring world can become an attainable goal for humanity.

Recognize opportunities to foster goodness in your life and act on them. Teach *and* learn about goodness from those around you; from spiritual beliefs, from your family and friends, from children, and from others you encounter. Commit to live with goodness in every aspect of life.

Getting back to good will allow goodness to flow through you into our world. From our collective differences to our fundamental similarities; from our unique, personal views and beliefs to the elements we share on a universal level, we are one and the same. No matter what our spiritual beliefs or status in society may be, we are bound to goodness and this life together. Now is the time for you to make a difference of goodness in your life, which in turn makes a difference of goodness for humanity and our world. In the end *there is right.*

Billions of Ways to Bring Goodness Into Our World, One Person at a Time

More than six billion people awaken every day on Earth, and each new dawn brings a gift of renewed opportunity for us to foster goodness toward nature and our fellow human beings. While goodness is encouraged and upheld every day by countless people around the world within every culture, creed, and society, billions of people corrode it with varying degrees of negative and selfish thoughts and actions. No one can exclusively pass the blame onto others for the selfishness and negativity that exists, because every person takes part in some way, at some time, in contributing to a less than desirable world, and is therefore responsible for improving it.

Imagine the possibilities…

We, all of us, are responsible for living with goodness. Whatever community or country we are a part of, regardless of personal lifestyles, beliefs, or opinions, each of us can do our part to collectively strengthen the human spirit of goodness. Simple thoughts and actions can bring our world back to good more than six billion times a day, and the potential is exponential when each of us takes part in the effort. Peace, compromise, prosperity, fulfillment, and happiness are the potential harvest when we find and travel unique paths to the common goal of true goodness. Let's work to...

get Back to Good!

CHAPTER 12

INSPIRATIONS

Here are some poems and quotes that have inspired me over the years, and continue to do so on a daily basis. I hope they inspire and motivate you, as well.

The greatest joy . . . . Giving
The ugliest personality trait . . . . Selfishness
The most satisfying work . . . . Helping Others

The most destructive habit . . . . Worry
The worst thing to be without . . . . Hope
The greatest problem to overcome . . . . Fear
The greatest asset. . . . . Faith

The greatest loss . . . . Loss of Self-Respect
The most prized possession. . . . . Integrity
The most worthless emotion. . . . . Self-Pity
The most contagious spirit . . . . Enthusiasm

The world's most powerful computer . . . . The Brain
The most crippling disease of failure. . . . . Excuses
The two most power-filled words . . . . I Can !
The two most difficult words to say . . . . I'm sorry

The deadliest weapon . . . . The Tongue

The greatest 'Shot in the Arm' . . . . Encouragement

The most dangerous pariah . . . . .A Gossip

The most helpful thing to do . . . . Forgive

The most powerful force in life. . . . . Love

The most beautiful attire . . . . .A Smile

The most effective sleeping pill. . . . . Peace of Mind

The strongest channel of communication . . . . .Prayer

The meaning of life: To believe, connect, love, share, and help one another.

–Unknown

Inspiring Quotes

"You cannot do a kindness too soon, for
you never know how soon it will be too late."

—Ralph Waldo Emerson

"We must not, in trying to think about how we can make a
big difference, ignore the small daily differences we can make,
which, over time, add up to big differences that we often cannot
foresee."

—Marian Wright Edelman

"Unless we think of others and do something for
them, we miss one of the greatest sources of happiness."

—Ray Lyman Wilbur

"To put the world right in order, we must first put the nation
in order; to put the nation in order, we must first put the family
in order; to put the family in order, we must first cultivate our
personal life; we must first set our hearts right."

—Confucius

"It is not what we take up, but
what we give up, that makes us rich."

—Henry Ward Beecher

"Hungry not only for bread — but hungry for love. Naked not only for clothing — but naked for human dignity and respect. Homeless not only for want of a room of bricks — but homeless because of rejection."

—Mother Teresa

"If you have much, give of your wealth; if you have little, give of your heart."

—Arabian Proverb

"Look to your health; and if you have it, praise God; and value it next to a good conscience; for health is the second blessing we mortals are capable of…"

—Izaak Walton

"Not he who has much is rich, but he who gives much."

—Erich Fromm

"I have one life and one chance to make it count for something… I'm free to choose what that something is, and the something I've chosen is my faith. Now my faith goes beyond theology and religion and requires considerable work and effort. My faith demands— this is not optional—my faith demands that I do whatever I can, wherever I am, whenever I can, for as long as I can, with whatever I have, to try to make a difference."

—Jimmy Carter

"You must be the change
you wish to see in the world."

—Gandhi

"How lovely to think that no one need wait a moment, we can start now, start slowly changing the world. How lovely that everyone, great and small, can make their contribution…how we can always, always give something, if only kindness."

—Anne Frank

"Life's most urgent question is:
What are you doing for others?"

—Dr. Martin Luther King, Jr.

"All people have a basic decency and goodness. If they listen to it and act on it, they are giving a great deal of what it is the world needs most. It is not complicated, but it takes courage. It takes courage for people to listen to their own good."

—Pablo Casals

"To work for the common good is the greatest creed."

—Woodrow Wilson

"Everyone who is seriously interested in the pursuit of science becomes convinced that a spirit is manifest in the laws of the universe—a spirit vastly superior to man, and one in the face of which our modest powers must feel humble."

-Albert Einstein

"You make a living by what you get,
but you make a life by what you give."

—Winston Churchill

"There was a time I used to reject those who were not of my faith.
Now my heart has grown capable of taking on many forms: a
pasture for gazelles, a convent for Christians, a temple for idols, a
Kaaba for the pilgrim, a table for the Torah, a book of the Koran.
My religion is love - whichever the route love's caravan shall take,
that path shall be the path of my faith."

-Muhyiddin Ibn 'Arabi

"Gratitude is not only the greatest of
virtues, but the parent of all the others."

—Marcus Tullius Cicero

"No good act performed in the world ever dies. Science tells us that
no atom of matter can ever be destroyed, that no force once started
ever ends: it merely passes through a multiplicity of ever-changing
phases. Every good deed done to others is a great force that starts an
unending pulsation through time and eternity. We may not know
it, we may never hear a word of gratitude or recognition, but it
will all come back to us in some form as naturally, as perfectly, as
inevitably, as echo answers to sound"

-William George Jordan

"Science is not only compatible with
spirituality, it is a profound source of spirituality."

—Carl Sagan

*It is not what they profess, but
what they practice that makes them good.*

—Greek Proverb

*"The welfare of each is
bound up in the welfare of all."*

—Helen Keller

*"The world is my country,
and my religion is to do good."*

—Thomas Paine

*I am only one, but still I am one;
I cannot do everything, but still I can do something;
And just because I cannot do everything,
I will not refuse to do the something that I can do.*

—Helen Keller

*"Everyone comes from the same source. If you
hate another human being, you're hating part of yourself."*

—Elvis Presley

*Faith is the strength by which
a shattered world will emerge into the light.*

—Helen Keller

"Religions are many and diverse,
but reason and goodness are one."

—Elbert Hubbard

"Never let the future disturb you.
You will meet it, if you have to,
with the same weapons of reason
which today arm you against the present."

—Marcus Aurelius

"Only a life lived for others is a life worthwhile."

—Albert Einstein

"Success consists of getting up just one more time than you fall."

—Oliver Goldsmith

"No one is born hating another person because of the color of his
skin, or his background, or his religion. People must learn to hate;
and if they can learn to hate they can be taught to love, for love
comes more naturally to the human heart than its opposite."

—Nelson Mandela

"If we really want to love,
we must learn how to forgive."

—Mother Teresa

"In helping others, we shall help ourselves, for whatever good we give out completes the circle and comes back to us."

—Flora Edwards

Do all the good you can,
By all the means you can,
In all the ways you can,
In all the places you can,
To all the people you can,
As long as ever you can.

—John Wesley

"Forgiveness helps you move forward. No one benefits more from forgiveness than the one who forgives."

—Unknown

"An apology is the superglue of life. It can repair just about anything."

—Lynn Johnston

"Kindness is the language which the deaf can hear and the blind can see."

—Mark Twain

We do not inherit the Earth from our ancestors, we borrow it from our children.

—Native American Proverb

5 Keys to Happiness:

1. *Free your heart from hatred*
2. *Free your mind from worries*
3. *Live simple*
4. *Give more*
5. *Expect less*

—Unknown

"There is no witness so terrible, no accuser so powerful as conscience which dwells within us."

—Sophocles

"When your intelligence don't tell you something ain't right, your conscience gives you a tap on the shoulder and says hold on."

—Elvis Presley

"I wanted to change the world - but I found that the only thing one can be sure of changing is oneself."

—Aldous Huxley

"As long as I can conceive something better than myself, I cannot be easy unless I am striving to bring it into existence."

—George Bernard Shaw

People will not always remember what you said;
People will not always remember what you did;
But people will always remember how you made them feel.

—Anonymous

The world is more malleable than you think
and it's waiting for you to hammer it into shape.

—Bono

"You will find, as you look back upon your life, that the moments that stand out are the moments when you have done things for others."

—Henry Drummond

"The greatest wealth is health."

—Virgil

Keep your dreams alive. Understand to achieve anything requires faith and belief in yourself, vision, hard work, determination, and dedication. Remember all things are possible for those who believe.

—Gail Devers

The Essence of a New Day

This is the beginning of a new day. You have been given this day to use as you will. You can waste it or use it for good. What you do today is important because you are exchanging a day of your life for it. When tomorrow comes, this day will be gone forever; in its place is something that you have left behind…let it be something good.

—Author Unknown

"Take the first step in faith. You don't have to see the whole staircase, just take the first step."

—Dr. Martin Luther King, Jr.

"If I have been of service; if I have glimpsed more of the nature and essence of ultimate good; if I am inspired to reach wider horizons of thought and action; if I am at peace with myself; it has been a successful day."

—Alex Nobel

The Critic

"It is not the critic who counts, nor the man who points out how the strong man stumbled or where the doer of deeds could have done them better. The credit belongs to the man who is actually in the arena, whose face is marred by dust and sweat and blood; who strives valiantly, who errs and comes short again and again, who knows the great enthusiasm, the great devotions, and spends himself in a worthy cause; who at the best knows in the end the triumph of high achievement, and who at the worst, if he fails, at least fails while daring greatly so that his place shall never be with those cold and timid souls who know neither victory nor defeat."

—President Theodore Roosevelt

Make Your Difference!

The ability to make a difference in your life, the life of another person, and the state of our world is always within reach. Find ways you can share: mentor a child, give time and money, show patience with friends and family, sign up as an organ donor, or reach out to offer assistance to those in need.

To assist in bringing more goodness into our world, I have created a non-profit website, www.makeyourdifference. org. You can find hundreds, even thousands of ways to help yourself and others. Please read the following press release to learn more.

LAKE VILLA, IL –Maybe solving the world's problems isn't easy; but Ken Ferrara believes pointing out the direction to a solution is.

"The solution is us — all of us — and I aim to show people how they can get involved in making the world a better place," said Ferrara, an Illinois man who is dedicated to positive networking through his web site, MakeYourDifference.Org.

MakeYourDifference.Org is a non-profit site whose name means what it says — providing ways for people make their difference. It is the concrete manifestation of Ferrara's book, *Getting Back to Good*.

"We've got to get back to doing good," Ferrara said. "We can complain all we want about the environment, poverty, hunger, health, and the state of our world today, but many of those problems can be solved by us. The idea behind Make Your Difference.Org is to inspire, engage, and connect people who realize they can be the solution, with organizations that are up and running, with proven track records at tackling life's problems."

Visitors will find scores of inspirational messages as well as links to charities, organizations and movements dedicated to the common good, that have one thing in common: they want to help.

MakeYourDifference.org includes links to sites to everything from animal rights to environmental issues to improving education and individual health. It includes sections for children and parents, crisis hot lines and links to special needs foundations.

"It's our job here to become a bulls eye for those folks who will learn they can connect to someone interested in solving their problem or, better yet, by helping them solve a problem near and dear to their heart and those they love," Ferrara said.

Perhaps best of all, MakeYourDifference.Org doesn't put limits on how someone can give something good to the world. Its links include charities, but visitors to the site will find countless ways they can give of their time, in a material manner or spiritually as well.

"We don't concern ourselves with what you want to give or how you want to give it. We just want to help you share it – to get back to doing the good that is in your heart," Ferrara said. "That means there are at least six billion potential solutions to any one problem, and I'll take those odds any day."

Make Your Difference.Org

Please visit MakeYourDifference.org to learn, earn, give, and become inspired. You can find and offer to help in these categories, as well as many more:

- Fight Hunger & Poverty
- Help & Care for Children
- Volunteer!
- Give Your Voice
- Fight Violence & Abuse
- Give Environmentally
- Give Tolerance
- Give and Find Health
- Raise Funds and Awareness
- Faith-Based Giving
- Help Yourself
- Family & Friends
- Give Kindness
- Resources for Parents and Kids
- Care for Animals
- Education
- Give Financially
- Special Needs
- CARE
- HOPE
- PEACE
- Honor Heroes

- Give Forgiveness
- Earn Free Money for Charity
- Sign up for our free newsletter
- Add your favorite organization or cause!

FROM THE AUTHOR

*"I wanted to change the world –
but I found that the only thing one
can be sure of changing is oneself."*

–Aldous Huxley

I like to quote the statement above when people ask me what inspired me to write this book. I was tired of the negativity and pessimism in my life as well as in the world at large. I noticed people were mean, impatient, and intolerant. Violence, greed and selfishness seemed to be prevalent everywhere I looked, leading me to ask, "Why can't we show more kindness and be more giving, trusting, grateful, and understanding? Why do people (myself included) have to be selfish and negative?"

I remember thinking about the state of our world — how negative it can seem at times, and I honestly felt I did my fair share to help out. You know what? I did do my fair share — my share of negativity and pessimism. It wasn't until years of separation from my family that I slowly became aware of the fact that the responsibility for much of the negativity I witnessed in the world, at work, and in my family was my own. Trapped in a downward spiral of negativity, I was often angry, resentful, ungrateful, and selfish.

My motto was, "What's in it for me?" If something did not directly affect or pertain to me, then it was someone else's problem. I was so wrapped up in an "all about me" attitude that I could not see the way I perceived and treated others lacked goodness — that I was treating people in the very ways I found so disheartening. The words I, me, my, and mine were used much too often in everyday encounters, and self-centered, intolerant behavior served to drain positive energy and joy from my life. My actions caused personal relationships to suffer, creating damaging rifts in my family, social, and professional lives.

- **Here's a glimpse into what brought me to where I am today.**

"A baby girl," shouted the Doctor, as he hurriedly passed my little daughter to the nurse anxiously waiting to perform the routine tests that newborns receive. I looked at my girlfriend, Jen. She was exhausted and pale after thirteen hours of labor but managed to crack a smile. I stroked her hair and gave her a kiss on the cheek. "We did it babe," I whispered, trying to show more confidence than I was feeling. We were young, scared, and excited at the same time.

The year was 1994. We had been dating for just over 5 years, but now life was forcing some huge, life-changing adjustments on us — the baby's cries constantly reminded us of that fact. We were relatively young at 21 years old, but decided we were going to make it. I quit my last year of college and took a job with the local phone company, while Jen would stay home with our baby. Thankfully, my parents invited us to live in my old bedroom until we got on our feet because the

$7.43 an hour paid to me by Ma Bell's offspring was making money a little tight.

Within a year, we were out in an apartment and doing our best to get by. Daily life encouraged and reminded us to press on, as we always tried to remain aware and thankful for our many blessings, and planned to get married soon. As life became busier, time went by and years passed. Before we knew it, our daughter was two years old. Throughout that time, however, things changed between us. There was awkward tension in the air when Jen and I spent time together, and our relationship just didn't feel the same. Maybe it was due to our hectic schedules, me working days and Jen working nights and weekends. Or, perhaps that feeling was coming from somewhere deep within myself.

By 1997, I had let myself go physically, and to be perfectly honest, I focused selfishly on myself. In doing so, my outlook on life, my mood, and my abilities were affected negatively. I was always tired and crabby, pushing away those closest to me and causing relationships to strain. Jen and I ended up splitting up for three long years, putting our precious daughter through hell.

Thankfully, over time and with the motivation and personal success of completing a physique transformation contest in Muscle Media Magazine (run at the time by Bill Phillips, author of *Body for Life*) I turned my life around. I started to realize that *I* was responsible for an abundance of negativity due to my selfish choices and perspectives, and only *I* could control the attitudes and actions that could bring about positive change.

Following years of stubborn selfishness, and the pain, self-pity, and unhappiness it produced, I began to ask, "Why am I so mean and negative at times? Why do I consider my needs to be more important than the needs of others? What can I do to bring more happiness and fulfillment into my life? How can I become a better person, both for myself, as well as for the people around me?"

I woke up to the fact that in order for this world to change, I must be the one to change. Of course, saying I would stop thinking and acting negatively is much easier said than done. But goodness, in all of its facets and dimensions, brings about such powerfully positive, productive results that I simply had to try my hardest to change for the better — you only get what you give.

From 1997 through 1999, I reached some low and scary points in life. I was separated from the ones I loved, depressed, and angry, and even in trouble with the law. At times I felt like I was out on an island – alone. To borrow from John Donne, I now understand that "no man is an island." Eventually, I overcame much of the negativity and pessimism in my life by using the ideas and processes in this book, and made getting back to good health a priority. By 2000 Jen and I had reconciled and were married in early 2001.

To be perfectly honest, I still struggle to follow the very advice and instruction on these pages because life can be hard. I have some difficult relationships in my family, and sometimes must work really hard to see my life's glass as half full. Choosing to be good is simply tougher than me at times, but I've learned to trust that life is a journey; a daily process with ups and downs, with bright lights and pitch blackness.

Different situations and challenges all serve in some way to help us learn to choose goodness to the best of our ability. Do I falter in this journey called life? Of course. Do I have to remove my shoe from my mouth? From time to time (okay, maybe a little more often than not). Overall, I can genuinely say working to get back to good empowers me to improve my perspective and enriches my relationships, my health, and my heart and soul. I'm sincerely and enthusiastically certain it can do the same for you.

The processes and techniques I've compiled here are the combined result of some of my life experience coupled with the wisdom imparted by those people who consistently embody the best attributes of the human spirit. I have assembled knowledge and lessons learned from personal struggles, hardships, and times of joy, as well as from examples of countless people who have shown the true goodness we are capable of, into something tangible — something that can help resolve questions, uncertainties, and challenges of life.

You can get back to good health with proper lifestyle changes and by incorporating healthy eating and exercise habits into your every day routines. (This was a very important step in my journey, which incidentally is one major reason I started writing.) Improving relationships by apologizing to others and forgiving, as well as maintaining a sense of gratitude and having faith, no matter what life throws your way are essential to getting back to good. Much of this book is the direct result of life experience, but I also drew on the strength people maintain through dark and dire challenges life thrust upon them, as well as the fundamental goodness so many people give out on a daily basis.

Getting back to good has the potential to make every day a better day. Of course, as I mentioned earlier, life isn't a fairy tale – hardships and challenges will still exist, but faith, positive focus, and guidance can help you find the goodness and happiness that is available for you to enjoy and share. My most sincere hope is to inspire you to focus on the positive and bring balance to your life. By presenting ways and techniques to become more kind, caring, compassionate, and grateful; by noticing all you are given everyday, I hope you will find and enjoy all the truly rich and fulfilling benefits living with goodness brings. All my best wishes for you…

~ About this Book ~

You won't find complicated comparisons of differing cultures or religions on these pages, as this book was written to be accessible and beneficial to people of all backgrounds and faiths. I hold extreme reverence for the multitude of differing beliefs in our diverse world because everyone travels a personal journey in life and has unique experiences and perspectives.

My most heartfelt wish is to respect your views, while offering you the positive, powerful, and practical values getting back to good can provide. To that end, I made every attempt to express ideas and messages in ways that do not detract from particular beliefs, while at the same time offering a straightforward guide to live with the goodness and tolerance that is applicable to everyone.

I am the first to admit you won't find any astonishing revelations, earth-shattering insights or complex philosophies between these covers. Many of the ideas expressed are as old as time, and I do not claim to present any new, fundamental beliefs or ideas that have not been written about, thought of, or discussed before. However, keep in mind that the information on these pages, from fundamental concepts to age-old knowledge, ultimately relates to our common link to goodness. The responsibility for living with goodness encompasses and applies to all people equally, no matter race, creed, or country.

Read with an open, optimistic mind, and keep the context of this book in the biggest picture possible. If you feel living with goodness does not apply to you, perhaps you will think differently when drawing your last breath. If you believe getting back to good is too idealistic to foster any meaningful change in our world, then I challenge you to take the energy of that negative perception, put it into thoughts and actions of goodness instead, and see what happens next.

From calling someone you have lost touch with to smiling at the person next to you, to making up with your siblings (I'm trying hard), *every* good thought and action will help bring our world back to good. Life is too short to wait for the next person to do it; take it upon yourself to be that next person—and pass it on.

"As long as I can conceive something better than myself, I cannot be easy unless I am striving to bring it into existence."

–George Bernard Shaw

My Debts of Gratitude

Thank God...

for giving all through many names, forms, words, interpretations, and faces. I understand and accept each day we see another sunrise as a gift, not something that is earned or even deserved. I am forever thankful for our ability to know, the power to love, the beauty of nature, and for the miracle of life.

To my wife,

Thanks for your constant support and encouragement. Through the years you helped me keep pen to paper and motivated me even when I pushed away. If not for you, my thoughts would still be scribbled onto scraps of paper instead of helping us. Thanks for your insight, endless patience in our apartment, and your ability to understand me. I love you.

To my kids,

Thanks for your stern hand in making sure I would finish — and for keeping our secret. You sacrificed many things because Dad was always "working on the book." You waited so patiently through my mood swings and procrastination, and took many, many trips to Great America with Mom until this final copy was ready. Well, here it is G, Bri, and T. Now we can practice basketball, fly kites, and build snowmen. I love you guys.

To my parents,

Thanks for your help over the years, your faith in me through all of my trials and mistakes, and for the countless hours you sat by my side, encouraging me. Although I was often the "Jack" of the family, the lessons I learned helped me understand and know. In this little paragraph, I cannot begin to express my gratitude to you for the love, compassion, and generosity you have shown me, especially to you Mom. Love, Ken

To my grandparents,

To Busia, Dziadzio, and Grammy: Thank you so much for your love and generosity. I will always carry your love and patience in my heart and soul. I am forever thankful for what you have given me and for what you continue to teach. I could not have completed this book without your help (especially recently, Busia). Love, Kenosha, Kenoosh, Animal.

For the rest of my family,

Auntie; Jim, Karen and family; Gary, Dawn, and family; Sal, Joyce and family, Licha and family; Keith, Alice and family; Tom, Michelle and family. To Mike (Big Stix), Martha and Family; Jimmy, Julie, and family; To Avelline (for your insightful advice and support); To Kurt and Tara, Jes, Christine, Aaron and Gina, as well as to the rest of my close friends and family who are equally important, thank you for giving me the insight, knowledge, and experience I needed in order to complete this book. To Mike, Anita and family, and Renee and Joe, through our share of disagreements and differing views, you have allowed me to see more clearly what living with goodness truly means.

And one big Thank you to Bill Phillips,

Bill, thanks for all you do to motivate and help people strive to become their best. You have helped me 'cross the abyss' two times now, and I am better because of you. Your kindness and sincerity works wonders, and I just want to say thanks.

Your friend,   Ken

Getting Back to Good To-Do Lists Summary

✓ Connecting With Goodness

❑ **Connect with goodness:**
  - ➤ Choose to accept the responsibility to live with goodness.
  - ➤ Do not cause harm, be intolerant, act selfishly, or foster hatred, *especially* in the name of a spiritual belief.
  - ➤ Negotiate any perceived problems in life with the courage faith provides.

❑ **Realize the purpose of spirituality:**
  - ➤ To connect with goodness.
  - ➤ Focus on being thankful.
  - ➤ Think and act with selflessness.
  - ➤ Have faith.

❑ **If you choose a spiritual connection of faith, focus on the true message of your beliefs:**
  - ➤ Be thankful, practice your faith in earnest, act kindly, and live with tolerance.
  - ➤ Do not focus on material aspects and specific practices of a spiritual belief to the point where you are not promoting goodness.

❑ **Become tolerant of differing spiritual views.**

➢ Understand that different religions, belief systems, and personal views come in many styles, shapes, and sizes, in order to fit the different, dynamic needs and circumstances of humanity.

➢ Illuminate the basic meaning of faith by showing tolerance of differing beliefs.

➢ Learn about and respect different beliefs to avoid spiritual tunnel vision.

✓ Look Up — Being Thankful

❑ **Be thankful for each new day:**
   ➢ Remember that every day is a gift — for you personally, as well as for the world.

❑ **Are there some tragedies or hardships that you have undergone and become stronger?**
   ➢ Use your experience as a foundation for helping someone else going through a similar challenge.

❑ **Be thankful for your health:**
   ➢ Remember that health is ultimately not in your hands.

❑ **Be thankful for your abilities:**
   ➢ Realize your abilities are gifts.
   ➢ Be humble as you remember accomplishments are not completely yours.

❑ **Remove obstacles that hinder a thankful perspective.**

❑ **Stop taking things for granted:**
   ➢ Consciously think about and be grateful for what is in your life every day.
   ➢ Show gratitude in thought as well as action.

➢ Recognize that you are not entitled to health, happiness, or a good life—they are gifts.

➢ Be thankful for, and humbled by the gifts you receive.

❑ **Be willing to accept that adversity may strike at any time in life.**

❑ **Be thankful through tough times.**

➢ Always find something to be thankful for, no matter what situation you are going through.

➢ Find thankful ways to deal with tough situations.

❑ **Do not pity yourself because of circumstances in life:**

➢ View life with thankfulness instead of pity.

➢ Do not compare your problems with the problems of others.

➢ Remember, your situation could always be worse.

➢ View adversity as something that will make you stronger.

➢ Be happy for others when good fortune embraces them.

❑ **Try not to worry about what cannot be controlled:**

➢ Much of life is beyond your control.

➢ Do not get so caught up with the details of life that you forget to act with thankfulness and goodness.

➢ Convert the energy spent on worrying into thankful thoughts and actions.

❑ **Strengthen your thankful perspective.**

❑ **Create your "I am Thankful For:" checklist:**

➢ Reflect on and write down everything you should be thankful for, from a new day, to health, to the goodness of humanity.

➢ Review your checklist several times a day and add to it often.

➢ Establish a routine for daily gratitude.

❑ **Maintain an attitude of gratitude to the best of your ability:**

➢ Take heart in the fact that people have gone through terrible situations and have been able to maintain a thankful perspective. So can you!

➢ Share some of the gifts you receive with others.

➢ Remember that a life clouded with selfishness cannot maintain a thankful perspective.

❑ **Couple your thankful perspective with thankful actions of goodness.**

• Recommended Reading:
  • *The Gratitude Journal* by Jack Canfield

✓ Look Within to Change

❑ **Understand why selfishness exists:**

  ➢ Wired in the mind for physical survival.

❑ **Understand why selflessness exists:**

  ➢ Wired in the mind for higher levels of self-preservation that are as important as the physical aspects of survival, if not more so.

❑ **Encourage your selfless instincts.**

  ➢ Identify selfish thoughts and behaviors, large and small:

  ➢ Do not rationalize you are not selfish simply because you have not broken any laws or committed significant actions of selfishness.

  ➢ Recognize that selfishness covers everything from physically hurting someone, to intolerance, to stealing, to making fun of someone.

❑ **Selfishness can be changed:**

  ➢ Foster goodness by replacing selfishness with selflessness.

❑ **Make a personal to-do list to encourage selflessness:**

✓ Selfish to Selfless

❑ **Assess your thoughts and actions.**

❑ **Rate yourself on the selfish/selfless scale:**
  ➢ Get an objective opinion to help you identify what you need to work on.
  ➢ List your selfish behaviors, make a plan, and commit to become selfless.

❑ **Be selfless to the best of your ability.**

❑ **Do not judge others with respect to their possessions or lifestyle, as long as no hurt or harm is caused:**
  ➢ Recognize that everyone is accountable for his or her own lifestyle and actions.

✓ Practice Giving

❑ **Give personal tolerance:**
  ➢ Tolerate unique viewpoints, as long as they do not cause hate or harm.
  ➢ Be as tolerant of the shortcomings of others as you are of your own.
  ➢ Do not force your views or opinions on others.

❑ **Give spiritual tolerance:**
  ➢ Accept the fact that there are many different ways of connecting to goodness.
  ➢ Do not force your spiritual views upon others.
  ➢ Practice tolerance by remembering your spiritual preference is not correct for everyone.

❑ **Find ways to identify and stop your intolerance.**

❑ **Give help to others:**
  ➢ Offering help is one of the best things you can do in life.
  ➢ Offer help in many different and unique ways.
  ➢ Do not miss an opportunity to help someone — you will need help someday.

❑ **Give forgiveness to others:**
  ➢ Replace feelings of hurt and anger by forgiving.

➤ Forgive as a means to release grudges that take away from your ability to foster goodness.

➤ Give Type II forgiveness to help you offer Type I Forgiveness.

❑ **Give Kindness to others:**

➤ Allow the natural trait of kindness to surface and act with kindness in your daily life.

➤ Every kind action becomes grand because of the exponential potential for goodness it contains.

➤ Give with kindness.

❑ **Give Environmentally:**

➤ Do not waste precious natural resources.

➤ Find ways to help our environment.

❑ **Create your own To-Do list — Giving.**

❑ **Remember, *giving* is good**

➤ Giving fulfills you in fundamental ways that simply are not reachable by any other means.

❑ **Visit www.makeyourdifference.org to find more ways and means to give.**

- Recommended Reading:
  - *Giving: How Each of Us Can Change the World* by Bill Clinton

✓ <u>Nurture Yourself</u>

❑ **Improve and maintain physical health:**

➢ Make healthy choices and incorporate exercise into your daily routine.

➢ Care for medical conditions.

➢ Limit bad influences on the body.

➢ Seek help to maintain your physical health when necessary.

❑ **Improve and maintain spiritual health:**

➢ Strengthen spiritual health.

➢ Do not harm, hurt, or be intolerant of others.

❑ **Improve and maintain emotional health:**

➢ Control your emotions so they don't overrule your thoughts and actions.

➢ Stay positive in your focus on life.

➢ Help others maintain emotional health.

❑ **Improve your financial condition.**

➢ Make wise financial choices.

➢ If you need assistance, get advice, information, and a helping hand from family, friends, or professionals.

❑ **Clear your conscience:**

➢ Find and fix things that weigh upon the health of your conscience.

➢ Take action to resolve any issues you are responsible for — before it's too late.

❑ **Improve and maintain all aspects of health to the best of your ability.**

❑ **Use your health to foster goodness.**

❑ **List and work to clear your conscience pests.**

- Recommended Reading:
  - *Body for Life* by Bill Phillips
  - *Eating for Life*

✓ Finding Purpose

❏ **Define complete purpose for life:**
  ➢ Reflect on what complete purpose means.
  ➢ Identify and fulfill your needs.
  ➢ Incorporate goodness into your life to find meaning.

❏ **Understand that there is more than a material aspect to life:**
  ➢ Remember, you won't be worrying about material possessions or accomplishments on your deathbed.

❏ **Live with goodness by being selfless:**
  ➢ Selfless thoughts and actions, no matter how big or small, are what you will take with you.

❏ **Help fulfill your complete purpose by getting back to good:**
  ➢ Have faith.
  ➢ Connect to goodness.
  ➢ Be tolerant of the ways in which other people connect.
  ➢ Be thankful.
  ➢ Be selfless.
  ➢ Learn to give.
  ➢ Take care.
  ➢ Treat others as you want to be treated.
  ➢ Be Good.

Journal:

Journal your feelings, dreams, goals, and aspirations on the following pages. Have fun and make this journal an integral part of your journey back to good.

_____

_____

_____

_____

_____

_____

_____

_____

_____

_____

_____

_____

_____

_____

_____

_____

_____

_____

_____

_____

_____

_____

_____

_____

Journal:

Journal:

Journal:

Journal:

_____

_____

_____

_____

_____

_____

_____

_____

_____

_____

_____

_____

_____

_____

_____

_____

_____

_____

_____

_____

_____

_____

_____

_____

_____

_____

_____

Journal:

Journal:

Journal:

Journal:

Journal:

Journal:

Journal:

Journal:

Journal:

Journal:

Journal:

Journal:

Journal:

Journal:

Journal:

Journal:

Journal:

Definition:

Getting Back to Good (getting - bak - too - guud),
v.n. **1.** the choice one makes to be good: *I will commit to live
with more goodness.* **2.** the process by which a person connects
with goodness. **3.** to be tolerant of differing views and beliefs.
4. to achieve and maintain a perspective of thankfulness for
everything in life. **5.** the process by which a person recognizes
selfishness and turns it into selflessness. **6.** to give: *help, kindness,
tolerance, forgiveness, care for nature, patience, compassion,
thankfulness, etc.* **7.** to care for all aspects of health in order
to foster goodness to one's full potential. **8.** the process of
combining definitions 1–7 to find and fulfill complete purpose
for life. **9.** to simply get back to good.

Contact Info:

Did Back to Good help you?

I would love to hear from you regarding how you will get back to good. Here are some ideas and questions to get you started. Feel free to add your own!

- Has this book changed your perspective? If so, how?
- How have you incorporated the principles and ideas in the book with your beliefs and lifestyle?
- How do you plan to live with more goodness?
- Has *Back to Good* motivated you to volunteer additional time, tolerance, money, or kindness?
- How are you taking care? Have you been able to apologize to others and clear some of your conscience pests? Have you forgiven someone and improved your quality of life? Did you improve emotional, spiritual, or physical health in order to repair relationships and foster goodness?

- Do you offer more respect and care for nature and our environment?

Please reply at: www.gettingbacktogood.com, simply click on "Have You Read the Book?" at the bottom of the website page.

ORDER INFO:

Getting Back to Good can be purchased online at www.gettingbacktogood.com and ordered at finer bookstores everywhere!

Thanks for taking the time to read this book.
Let's all make a difference!

www.ingramcontent.com/pod-product-compliance
Lightning Source LLC
Chambersburg PA
CBHW061352280526
45784CB00001B/231